The acute poorly performing sport horse

The acute poorly performing sport horse

CESMAS 2008

edited by:

Arno Lindner

Arbeitsgruppe Pferd

Wageningen Academic Publishers

ISBN 978-90-8686-072-2

First published, 2008

Wageningen Academic Publishers
The Netherlands, 2008

Foreword

Great, CESMAS 2008 is taking place in Utrecht, Netherlands! The home of Marianne and many persons that I know pretty well by now. Almost like my home too! This is one of the bounties of organising international meetings!

The subject chosen to be tackled intensively in this conference is 'Acute Poor Performance in Sport Horses'. We all know that the determination of performance-limitation, is challenging. Even more when the next important competition is close. Information in literature on the subject is scarce or very general. Thus, the authors of the articles in this book were asked to write mainly about their experience. They have done a great job, to the extent that I feel that their information will be taken as reference and trigger the research on additional information and the compilation of available one. Thank you to all!

I am indebted very much to all members of the scientific committee. They have done a wonderful job in selecting the subjects and speakers for the conference and reviewing the submitted work. The expanded abstracts accepted – and whose authors were willing to publish them – are also in the book. Thank you to the authors!

I am very grateful to the responsible persons of our industrial partners! Early on they were willing to sponsor (again) the meeting. This 'support cushion' allows for much easiness!

I would like to wish readers pleasure reading the book.

Arno Lindner

Scientific Committee

Warwick M. Bayly, USA
Hilary Clayton, USA
Anne Couroucé-Malblanc, France
Jean-Marie Denoix, France
Sue Dyson, United Kingdom
Adriana Ferlazzo, Italy
Arne Holm, Norway
Arne Lindholm, Sweden
Arno Lindner, Germany
José Luis López Rivero, Spain
Marianne Sloet van Oldruitenborgh-Oosterbaan, Netherlands

Sponsors

Boehringer Ingelheim Vetmedica
Equine Veterinary Products
IDEXX
Vetoquinol / Equistro
Videomed
Equine Veterinary Journal
Intervet
TRT Nonvasiv
Vetray

In Memoriam Steven Wickler († May 2007)

Table of contents

Abstracts

Articles

What do we know about the poor performance horse?

Tatiana Art and Emmanuelle van Erck
Center of Equine Sports Medicine, Faculty of Veterinary Medicine, University of Liege, Belgium; tatiana.art@ulg.ac.be

What are the determinants of performance?

Basic considerations on exercise physiology

Horses are athletes able to achieve incredible performances in speed, height, power or endurance. Whatever the equestrian discipline considered, the accomplishment of a performance is the result of a complex physiological balance, long term adequate physical preparation, exterior circumstances, which include rider intervention, and the will of the equine athlete to push its limits. When considering the pure physical side of performance, the horse's outstanding athletic capability is related to their high maximal aerobic capacity (namely due to a high capillary and mitochondria density in muscles), their large intramuscular stores of energy substrates especially glycogen (140 mmol/kg of muscles vs 80-100 mmol/kg in man), their aptitude to increase oxygen carrying capacity related to spleen contraction (that release 50% of the total red blood cells) and the dramatic increase of their cardiac output during exercise.

Whatever the type of exercise performed, ATP is the basic energy molecule used to ensure muscular work. Synthesis of new ATP is therefore necessary to replace the expended ATP. In horses, as in every species, metabolic anaerobic pathways (alactid but especially lactid acid) may be used for brief periods (such as at the onset of exercise or when exercise intensity is superior to VO_{2max}) (Figure 1). Nevertheless, in the equine species, aerobic pathways (based on substrate oxidation – either carbohydrate or fatty acids) are the predominant way to synthesize ATP. While in human athlete running 100 m, 99% of the ATP are synthesized by the anaerobic pathways, in Thoroughbred horses running 1000 m, only 30% of ATP is provided by this way. Therefore, in horses, the accomplishment of an exercise depends on adequate substrates availability and, most of the time, on adequate oxygen supply (Eaton *et al.*, 1995) (Figure 2).

Oxygen transport from (1) the ambient air to the exchange zones in the lung, and (2), from the exchanging zone into the muscles mitochondria, is achieved by the coordinated action of the respiratory and cardiovascular systems. During exercise, the increase in metabolic rates imposes an increased load on all physiological steps involved in what is called the **oxygen chain** (Figure 3).

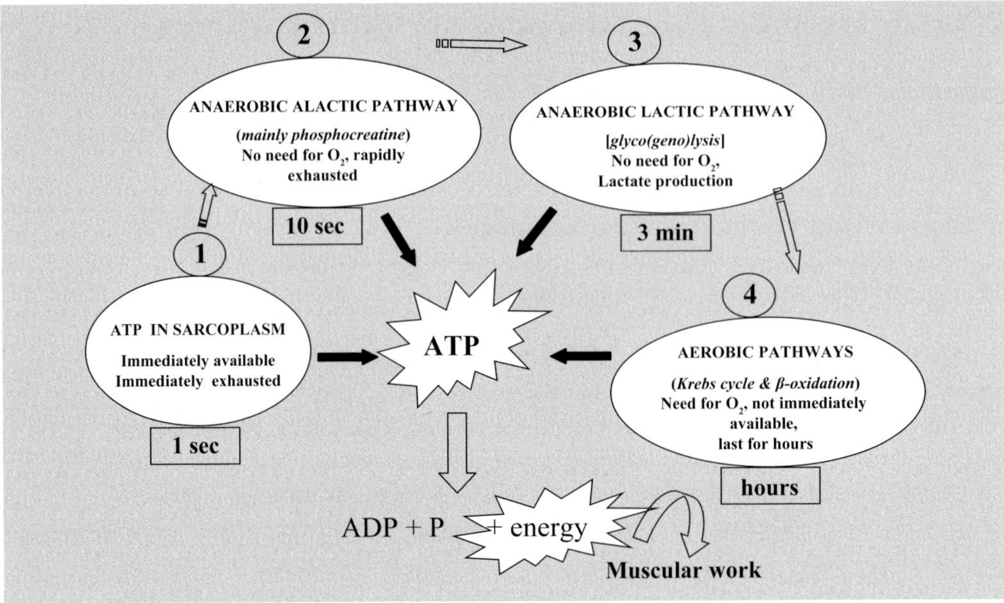

Figure 1. The different pathways of synthesis of ATP during exercise. Anaerobic ways provide ATP without oxygen: they are immediately available at the onset of exercise but rapidly exhausted. Aerobic pathway rests on substrate oxidation. At the onset of exercise, there is a delay before they are totally functional, but once available, they may synthesize ATP during several hours. If exercise intensity is high, their capacity of production may be exceeded and further ATP will be synthesized by the anaerobic lactic pathway.

The efficiency of the links of this chain may be modified by training or illness. The soundness and capacity of these systems will therefore play a substantial role in determining the performance potential of a horse. These steps are sequential and non duplicative: consequently a limitation in one of these steps will inevitably limit the efficiency of the whole chain.

> Identifying the weak link in the *oxygen chain* is one of the biggest challenges for the sports medicine practitioner.

Each discipline is associated to specific exercise-induced adjustments and/or troubles

During exercise, there is a coordinated response of all the body systems involved to increase energy availability, to maintain acid-base balance and to control body temperature. The nature of the physiologic response essentially depends on the exercise intensity and duration. Competitions as different as endurance riding (160 km) or racing (1500 m) present great differences in energy demands –

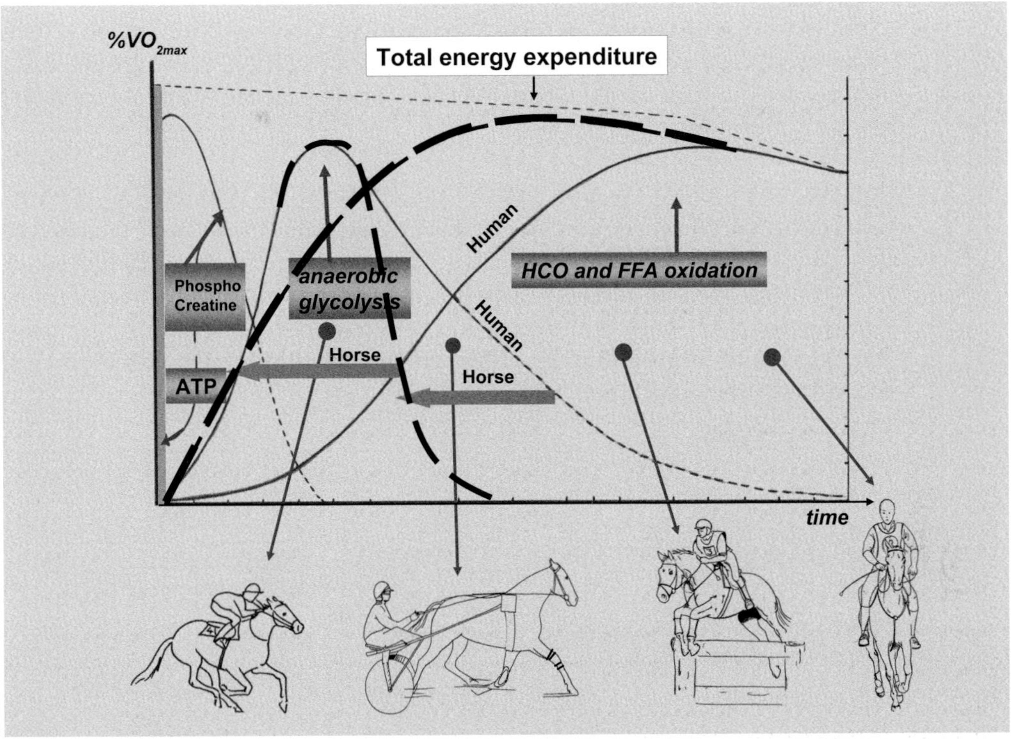

Figure 2. The relative contribution of the different pathways of synthesis of ATP in function of the discipline. Contrarily to what is reported for the human athlete, in the horse during high speed exercise, the aerobic pathway, ie oxidation of carbohydrate and free fatty acid, is the dominant way of ATP production. Performances in horses therefore mainly depend on adequate oxygen supply.

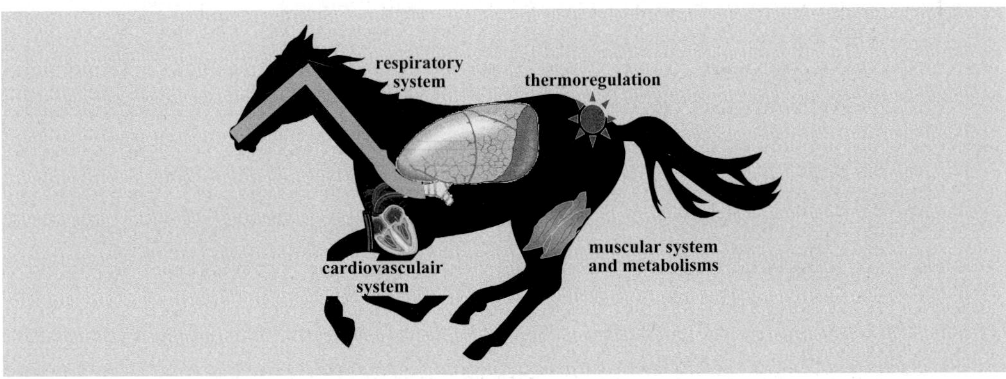

Figure 3. The oxygen chain during exercise: increase in minute ventilation and in alveolar ventilation, diffusion at the level of the alveolo-capillary membrane, cardiac output and oxygen-carrying capacity (splenic contraction), muscles blood distribution, oxygen diffusion into the muscles and use of oxygen by the muscular machinery.

high intensity effort results in a greater energy production from carbohydrates (muscles glycogen and blood glucose) while long lasting moderate intensity exercise (endurance races) favors the use of fat (Figure 4), biomechanical function, thermoregulation, etc...

High exercise intensity (gallop and trot racing) is mainly characterized by high blood acidosis. Why? Generally, when exercise intensity is high, lactate and associated H^+ is produced because of the partial use of anaerobic metabolism for ATP synthesis. Despite a certain buffering capacity (by proteins and bicarbonates) the presence of H^+ both in the muscular cells and in the blood, during intense exercise results in pronounced acidemia. The sometimes also observed CO_2 retention further contributes to this acidosis.

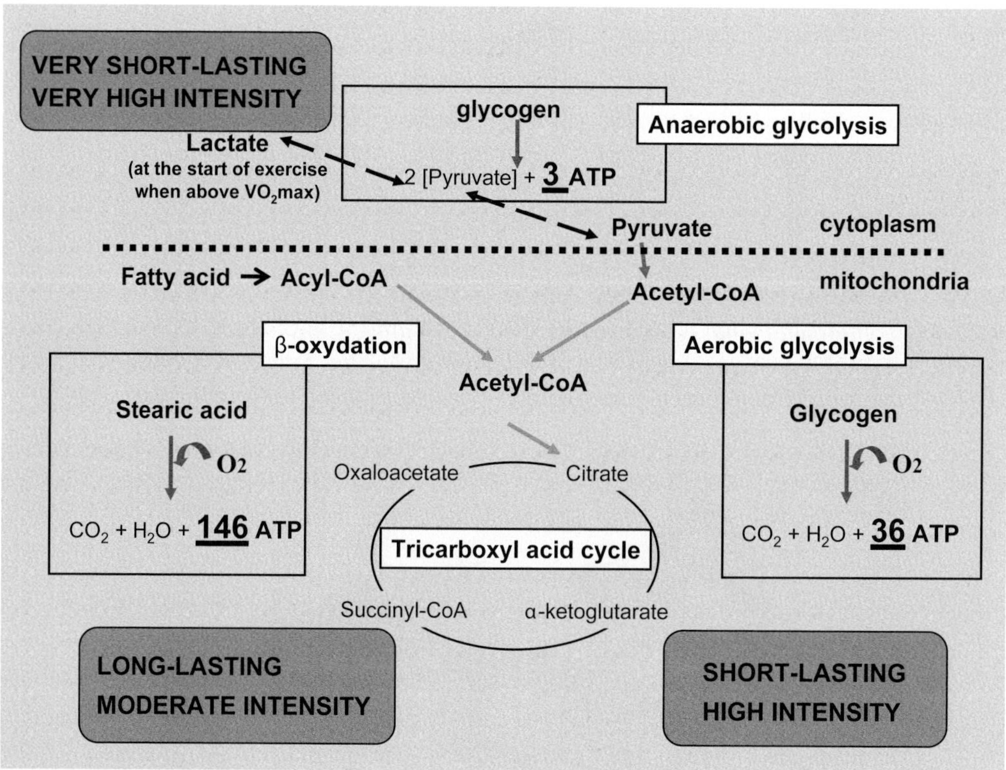

Figure 4. The final output in ATP production is dramatically different from one pathway to the other. The anaerobic glycolysis allows for the synthesis of only 3 ATP per mol of glycogen, while the complete oxidation of one mol of glycogen allows the synthesis of 36 ATP. Free fatty acids are by far the more efficient source of energy: the quantity of ATP produced is much more important and above all, only 30% of the energy liberated is lost as heat, which is low compared to the 70% heat lost with carbohydrate oxidation. This explains why in endurance, free fatty acids are preferentially used.

On the opposite, long lasting endurance race will rather result in hypochloremic alcalosis, together with dehydration and possibly hyperthermia. Why? Seventy five percent of the energy used during exercise is dissipated as heat, and exercise therefore induces significant raise in body temperature. The heat is transported from the muscles to the skin (and respiratory system) by the venous network and then dissipated at this level. Evaporation of sweat is the main way for heat transfer to the environment. It has been estimated that a racing endurance horse may lose 6-15 l/hour of sweat during 10 hours. Endurance horses may consequently lose substantial volumes of water and electrolytes. The system is efficient as long as the ambient temperature is lower than the body's temperature, the water saturation of ambient air is low and the horse is sufficiently hydrated to sweat adequately. Therefore, despite the fact that high intensity exercise may induce important increase in muscle, blood and body temperature, dehydration, electrolyte imbalance or heat shock are generally described in horses during prolonged exercise, namely in 3-day eventers and endurance horses.

The effects of training

Training or conditioning is a chronic repetition of exercise that induces physiological and morphological adaptations. Some tissues or functions are malleable and are significantly improved by training (muscles, cardiac function) but other remained unchanged (lung and respiratory function) (Figure 5). In general, among the adaptable systems, the soft tissues (skeletal and cardiac muscles for example) adapt rather rapidly while hard tissues (tendons and bones) take longer to improve.

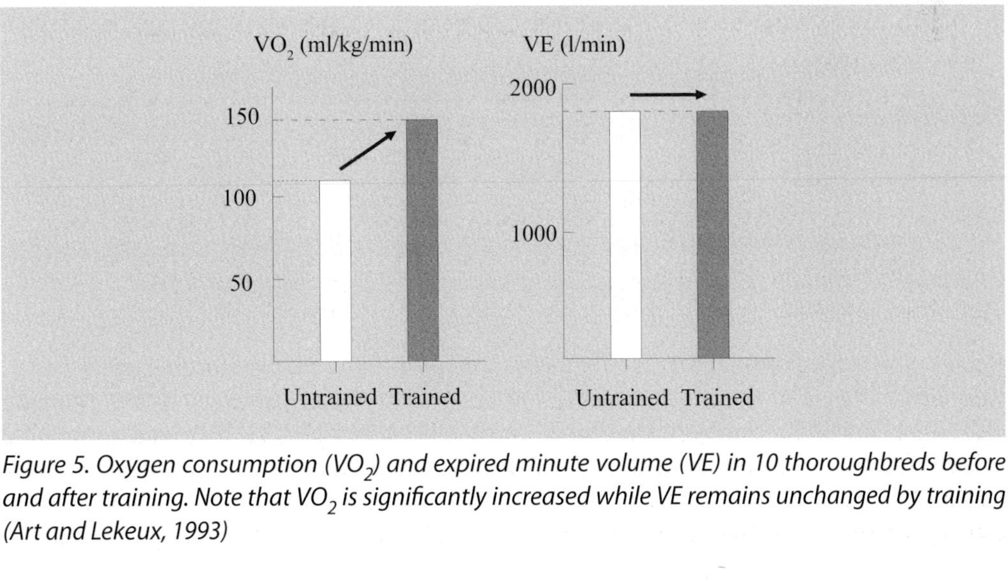

Figure 5. Oxygen consumption (VO_2) and expired minute volume (VE) in 10 thoroughbreds before and after training. Note that VO_2 is significantly increased while VE remains unchanged by training (Art and Lekeux, 1993)

Because the respiratory system is not anatomically enlarged nor functionally improved by training, it is likely to become the limiting factor to performance in well trained animals (Figure 6).

Factors limiting performance in healthy horses

The importance of the aerobic pathway in the muscular energetic supply, whatever the discipline, is well recognized in horses. However, speed race horses are probably mainly limited by the oxygen supply at the muscular level. Indeed, despite the large exchanging pulmonary area, the dramatic increase in pulmonary ventilation, the increase in cardiac output and packed cell volume, horses exercising at a level higher than 60% of VO_2max become hypoxemic, and even hypercapnic (Bayly *et al.*, 1983).

Numerous research studies have shown that horses possess a high muscle mass which has enormous metabolic requirements resulting in O_2 uptake and CO_2 production that exceed the ventilation capacities, especially in well trained horses. These observations strongly suggest that the respiratory system may be

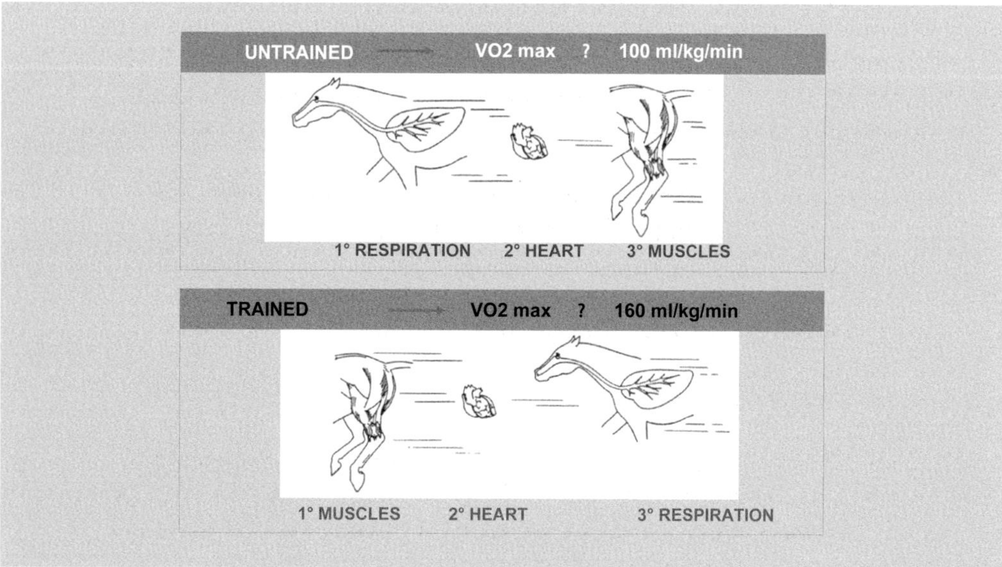

Figure 6. This figure illustrates the putative factors limiting maximal performance in healthy horses, according to fitness. In the untrained horse, the weak link of the oxygen chain is most probably muscle metabolism and development (size, proteins content, oxidative enzymatic machinery, capillarization…). The respiratory system is redundant. In the trained horse, the improvement of the muscles oxidative capacity is so important that the respiratory system, which remains unchanged, is unable to satisfy their O_2 needs.

the ultimate limiting factor to high intensity exercise in horses. In human athletes however, it would rather seem that it is the availability of O_2 in the muscles, ie diffusion and transport, which represents the limiting factor.

Some anatomic and physiologic peculiarities specific to the horse may explain the fact that respiration is the weak link of the oxygen chain.

1. Length, section and shape of the upper airway contribute to a high anatomical dead-space, and associated to the compulsory nasal breathing, result in an increased resistance to airflow and energetic cost of breathing, which probably 'down regulates' the increase in pulmonary ventilation during intense exercise.
2. Mixed venous blood coming back from the peripheral tissues (muscles) has a partial pressure in O_2 as low as 15 mmHg, which is in relation to the dramatic O_2 removal by the working muscles.
3. Impairment of gas diffusion at the level of the alveolo-capillary membrane because of the dramatic increase of cardiac output reduces the time for gas exchange. A relative impairment of the ventilation/perfusion ratio has been also suggested as a possible reason for the gas exchange impairment.

This limiting role of the respiratory system is probably more important in horses racing at high speed on short and middle distances than in horses racing on very short (quarter horses) or very long distances (endurance horses). As previously noted, performance of endurance horses will above all depend on their capacity to regulate their fluid and electrolytic homeostasis.

> The understanding of what phenomena are most likely to limit performance in healthy horses according to their discipline is important, especially in identifying the possible cause of poor performance.

What are the potential causes of poor performance?

What do we call poor performance?

Throughout the rest of this paper, a distinction will be made between poor performance and exercise intolerance. The latter syndrome is characterized by recent and obvious changes in the performance during competition – or even during training work – and is often related to the occurrence of a genuine and specific problem. Exercise intolerance is considered by the authors as different from poor performance, which generally means performance under expectations, and may be due to several reasons including poor genetic potential, inappropriate management, or simply excessive expectations of the owners (Figure 7).

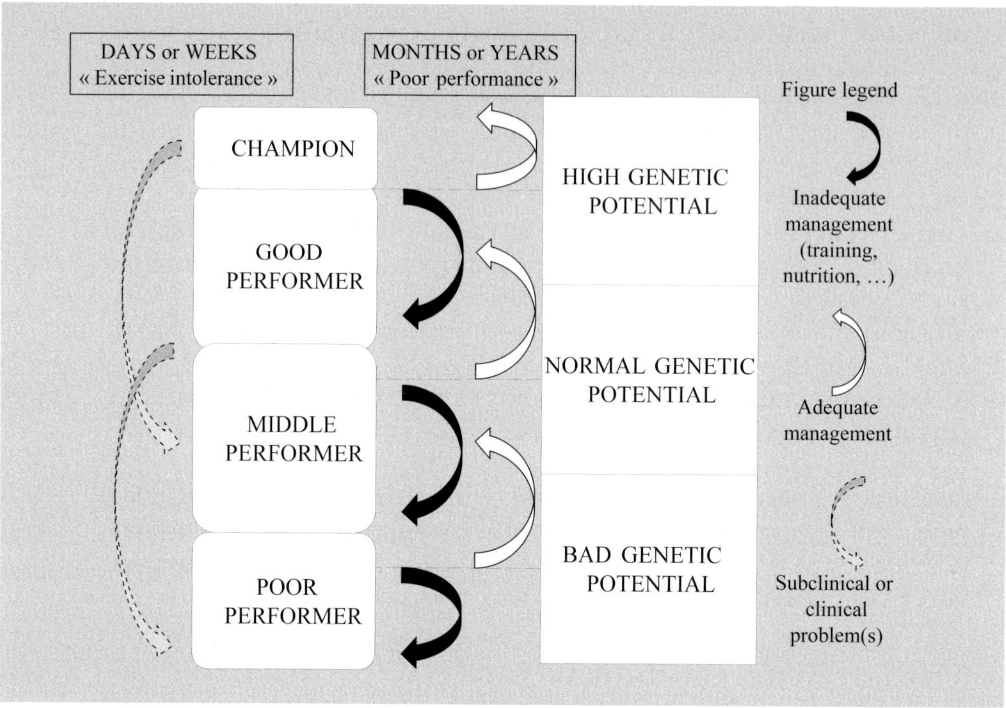

Figure 7. The determinants of performance and the possible causes for poor performance and for exercise intolerance.

While it is relatively easy to find the cause(s) of exercise intolerance with appropriate tests, it is generally more difficult to point out relevant (often multiple) causes of unsatisfactory performances in the poor performer.

Epidemiologic data from Sports Medicine Centers

Surprisingly, despite the fact that sports medicine has existed for more than 25 years, there are only 2 published retrospective studies on around 300 horses reporting statistics on the causes of poor performance (Morris and Seeherman, 1991; Martin *et al.*, 2000). Without doubt, the most commonly diagnosed reason for wastage is musculoskeletal injury. The locomotion problems are not presented in this review, which only focuses on the oxygen transport chain and muscles energetic. In both studies, examination of the horses was based on a thorough laboratory examination including echocardiography, treadmill test with video-endoscopy and electrocardiography, as well as pre- and post-exercise biochemistry

In the study of Martin *et al.* (2000), a definite cause of poor performance was identified in 256/348 (73.5%) horses. The causes of poor performance were distributed as follows: 148 upper airway dynamic obstructions (mainly dorsal displacement of the soft palate, dynamic pharyngeal collapse, idiopathic laryngeal hemiplegia), 22 combinations of upper airway obstruction and cardiac arrhythmias, 19 heart problems (decreased fractional shortening), 10 subclinical exertional rhabdomyolysis (increase of CK above 1000 IU/l after exercise), 15 lameness and 9 other disorders. These results were close to the results of the report of Morris and Seeherman in 1991. Surprisingly and for incomprehensible reasons, none of these 2 laboratories have performed lower airway examination nor tracheo-bronchial or broncho-alveolar lavage (BAL)! This may explain the 26.5% of horses remaining without reliable diagnosis in the study of Martin *et al.* (2000).

Other studies performed on smaller groups of racing horses (Couëtil and Denicola, 1999; Van Erck *et al.*, 2006), in which cytologic examination of BAL was included in the string of tests, reported the major incidence of lower airway subclinical problems (including Inflammatory Airway Disease -IAD-, Recurrent Airway Obstruction -RAO-, Exercise-Induced Pulmonary Hemorrhage -EIPH) on exercise tolerance.

It must be pointed out that this kind of information are sparse or nonexistent for jumping, event and endurance horses, and to the best of our knowledge not yet published.

Further remarks:

- None of the studies distinguished the poor performer from the exercise intolerant horses.
- None of the studies examined the stomach for presence of ulcers, which are frequently associated with poor performance.
- Some problems are found but it is difficult to establish if they are definitely the cause for poor performance (grade II/1 idiopathic laryngeal hemiplegia or EIPH for example).
- Cardiac murmurs are frequently heard but rarely have a functional impact.
- A non-negligible part of horses remain without definitive diagnosis.

At the Equine Sports Medicine Center of Liege, statistics have been made on the horses referred between 2000 and 2004 for exercise intolerance or poor performance (Figure 8). The distribution of the disciplines is different from the aforementioned studies: 50% of the horses examined are showjumping horses. These horses were examined at rest (clinical examination biochemistry, arterial blood gases, pulmonary function test by impulse oscillometry, upper airway endoscopy), during exercise (heart rate, ECG, lactate and endoscopy) and after

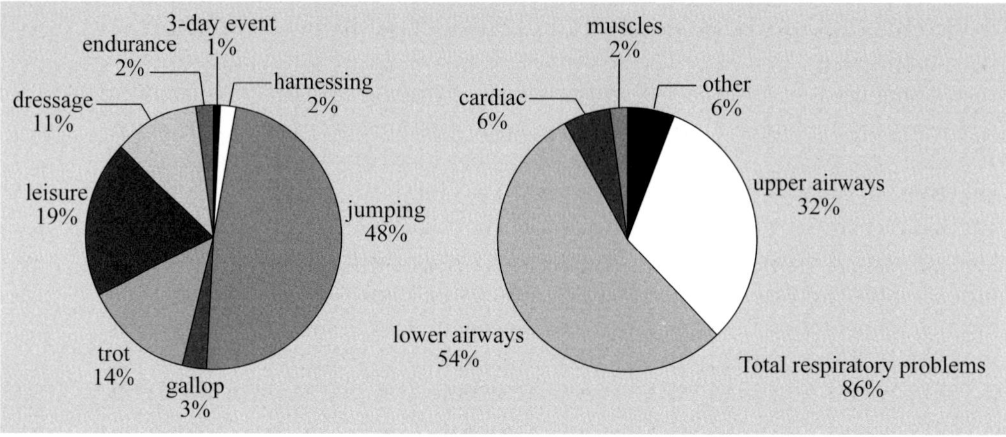

Figure 8. Repartition of 345 horses referred to the Center of Equine Sports Medicine of Liege between 2000 and 2004 for poor performance or exercise intolerance. Show jumpers represent half of the horses. Lower airway problem was the first diagnosis, followed by upper airway dysfunction (Van Erck et al., *2006).*

exercise (echocardiography, lower airway endoscopy and BAL, biochemistry). A diagnosis of lower respiratory problem was set out in 54% of the cases, mainly RAO, but also IAD. These statistics should however be considered with caution: (1) our laboratory is known to have a scientific expertise in chronic pulmonary diseases and this fact most probably induces a bias in the population of referred horses; (2) although 54% of all horses referred have been diagnosed as suffering from lower airway disease, the potential repercussion of these problems on the exercise capacity depends on the discipline and will be more harmful in race horses than in jumping horses.

In conclusion, apart from musculo-skeletal problems, respiratory problems (upper or lower airway diseases or often a combination of both conditions) are reported as being the main cause of poor performance and exercise intolerance in sports horses. Therefore upper airway endoscopy and BAL are essential complementary exams in the search of the cause for poor performance or exercise intolerance.

Systems that could potentially be responsible for decreased performance

As discussed in the previous chapters, all the systems involved in the oxygen chain may be the potential cause of exercise intolerance. A thorough presentation of each system as potential cause for exercise intolerance is given elsewhere in these proceedings and will be discussed by other speakers of this congress.

Therefore, this chapter will just enumerate the main problems encountered in sports medicine.

In all studies, whatever the sports discipline of the investigated horses or the method used, respiratory problems represent around half or more of the definitive cause of exercise intolerance or poor performance.

Because the respiratory system is the main factor limiting performance in healthy horses, any respiratory problem, even subclinical, will significantly impede athletic capacity. The lack of adaptation to training and the high prevalence of respiratory disease explain the important role of this system in the occurrence of exercise intolerance.

The foal is born with its intrinsic respiratory capability and the only event that may happen later is a decrease in its respiratory capability, for multiple reasons: housing in dusty environment and feeding with dry food, training, transportation, mingling during competition, all factors that favor the development of infectious, inflammatory and allergic diseases. Although the resistance of the lower airway account for only 20% of the total pulmonary resistance in healthy horses, when their lumen is narrowed by functional (mucus hypersecretion, bronchospasm), infectious (mucopus), or other problems (pulmonary hemorrhage, oedema, dynamic collapse), their resistance increases and becomes a factor limiting ventilation.

It is important to know that respiratory diseases can progress without overt clinical signs such as cough, nasal discharge. Owners may report that their horse lacks thrive during exercise or is difficult to condition without being aware of an underlying respiratory problem and ancillary exams such as airway endoscopy or sampling is necessary for the veterinarian to establish the diagnosis. It is therefore most likely that the prevalence of lower respiratory diseases remains currently underestimated.

Furthermore, the upper airways also contribute to the high prevalence of respiratory problems as cause of poor performances. To provide the lowest resistance due to friction and turbulence, the horse's upper airways should ideally have been short, large, straight and rigid. On the contrary, they are long, narrowed in bottleneck shaped parts as the larynx, changing of direction, namely at the level of the pharynx and the entrance in the lung, and compliant (ie most of the parts are soft tissues only sustained by muscles or cartilages and therefore susceptible to dynamic collapse when submitted to compressing transmural pressure). Moreover, the horse is unable to bypass the nasal cavities by breathing through the mouth. Knowing that resistance to airflow is inversely proportional to the radius exponent 4, one can understand the major effect on the resistance to airflow of a small reduction of the radius. This reduction or sub-obstruction may be due to functional, inflammatory or infectious problems.

Muscular problems, when diagnosed, are often subclinical or are responsible for poorly specific signs resulting in decreased performance. The diagnosis of exertional myopathy rests on the observation that the CK activity is more than doubled compared to the pre-effort resting values, from 30 minutes after exercise. For other authors, the post-exercise values are higher than 1000 iu/l in case of muscular problems.

Cardiac murmurs and arrhythmia are commonly detected in performance horses, creating a problem in the determination of their possible functional effects on exercise tolerance. Remember that the probability of a heart disease as a cause of poor performance is low. Arrhythmias such as AVB are without significance as long as they disappear at exercise. The main arrhythmias susceptible to affect performance are atrial fibrillation and ventricular premature systoles (VPS). Isolated VPS are rarely significant. If frequent, they may be related to a myocardial problem, but also to systemic troubles including electrolytic imbalance.

How to determine the cause(s) of poor performance?

At rest

History is an essential element to discriminate the poor performance horse from the horse suffering from sudden exercise intolerance.

Horses suffering from poor performance or exercise intolerance are often asymptomatic. However a thorough physical **examination** is essential, especially to decide the further tests and examination that should be used. Moreover, although in most of the cases, the problem is located in one of the systems involved in the pursuit of exercise, abnormalities in any of the body systems may also impair the performance.

Remember that, in horses, **lameness** is the first recognized reason for poor performance, temporary withdrawal from training or definitive retirement from competition. Therefore any gait irregularity, any pain at the level of the osteo-articular system should be considered as a potential cause of exercise impairement. Consequently, even if there is a doubt about the potential implication of another system (cardiac murmur, respiratory noise), lameness problems of any nature should be resolved before continuing ancillary examinations.

Blood biochemistry and arterial blood gas analysis will seldom help to diagnose the cause of poor performance but may help in exercise intolerance.

Performed before and/or after exercise, they may help to detect inflammatory or infectious problems, muscular disorders, relative anemia, dehydration, electrolytic imbalance.

Examination of the cardiac system involves examination of the peripheral perfusion and pulse, careful cardiac auscultation, ECG recording, and if possible, Doppler-echocardiography. Some significant morphological and functional problems can remain undiagnosed unless echocardiography is undertaken (myocardial dyskinesis, reduced fractional shortening, quiet valvular regurgitations,...).

Endoscopic examination of the upper airways (UA) should be performed in every horse suffering from exercise intolerance. Indeed, because of their anatomy and physiology, UA resemble a bottleneck within the respiratory tract. Therefore, any abnormality that would further reduce the narrow airway section would be a potential factor of impaired ventilation and consequently impaired performance. The lumen of the trachea should also be visualized to check for the presence of mucus or blood in the airway.

Pulmonary function tests (for example with the forced oscillation technique) may help to assess possible airway subobstruction and abnormal resistance to airflow (Figure 9).

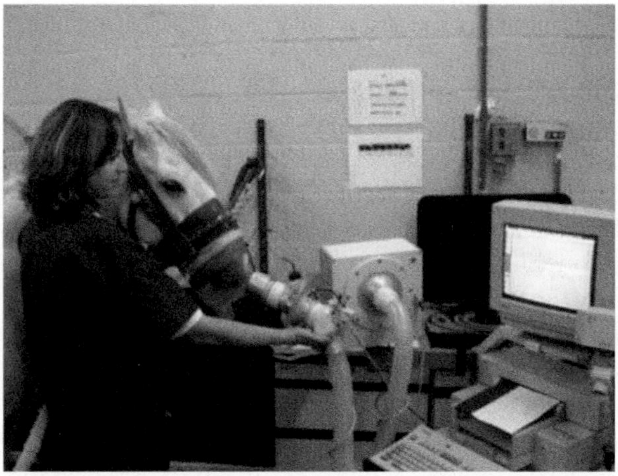

Figure 9. Pulmonary function test by the forced oscillation: this method is totally non invasive and well tolerated by the horses. It is more sensitive than the 'oesophageal balloon technique' and allows to differentiate problems at the level of the upper and lower airway.

Two remarks must be done: (1) Some findings could be insignificant because they have few if no impact on ventilation (pharyngeal hyperplasia, grade II/1 and II/2 laryngeal asymetry, short or flaccid epiglottis); (2) most of the problems occurring at the level of the UA are dynamic (ie they only become obvious when UA are submitted to large pressure changes during intense exercise). Consequently, observation of normal UA at rest is inconclusive and does not exclude the occurrence of abnormalities during exercise. Indeed, while most UA dynamic obstructions create respiratory noise during exertion, some can occur without associated noise, making diagnosis more challenging. Although, it is necessary to check the UA at rest, and without sedation, exercise-endoscopy is generally an essential complementary exam in poor performers.

During exercise

Blood lactate and heart rate may be measured during exercise. The main purpose of these measurements is to established curves of both values in function of speed and to interpolate VLA4 (ie the speed at which blood lactate is equal to 4 mmol/l) and V200 (ie the speed at which the heart rate equals 200 beats/min). Both values are likely to be indicators of aerobic capacity (VLA4 and V200) and cardiovascular capacity (V200) and generally used for the evaluation of fitness and state of training (Figure 10).

In some horses suffering from poor performance or exercise intolerance, the values may be out of range. The interpretation of this observation may be difficult: the horse may have limited intrinsic capability, may be inadequately trained or may really suffer from a problem. Consequently, the fact that measured parameters are abnormal should be first of all considered as a warning (Figure 11). These observations must be interpreted at the light of a detailed questionnaire on the horse's past and current performances, state of training and competing level, but also of the observations made during exercise (for example, a nervous horse may have higher lactate at low level of exercise than at high level). Taking this remarks into account, they can be used as a tool to help determine the origin of poor performance and/or to prioritize the investigation of certain problems and/or to estimate the repercussion of these problems on the onset of fatigue.

Electrocardiography during exercise, with a telemetric or a recording holter systems may help to identify cardiac arrhythmias such as paroxysmal atrial fibrillation and salves of VPC (Figure 12). Exercise level should be sufficient to elicit potential cardiac rhythmic problems. Cautions must be taken when interpreting cardiac rhythm within minutes of cardiac slowing after exercise in athletic horses. Transient post-exercise sinus arrhythmia is a normal finding that does not indicate any cardiac pathology.

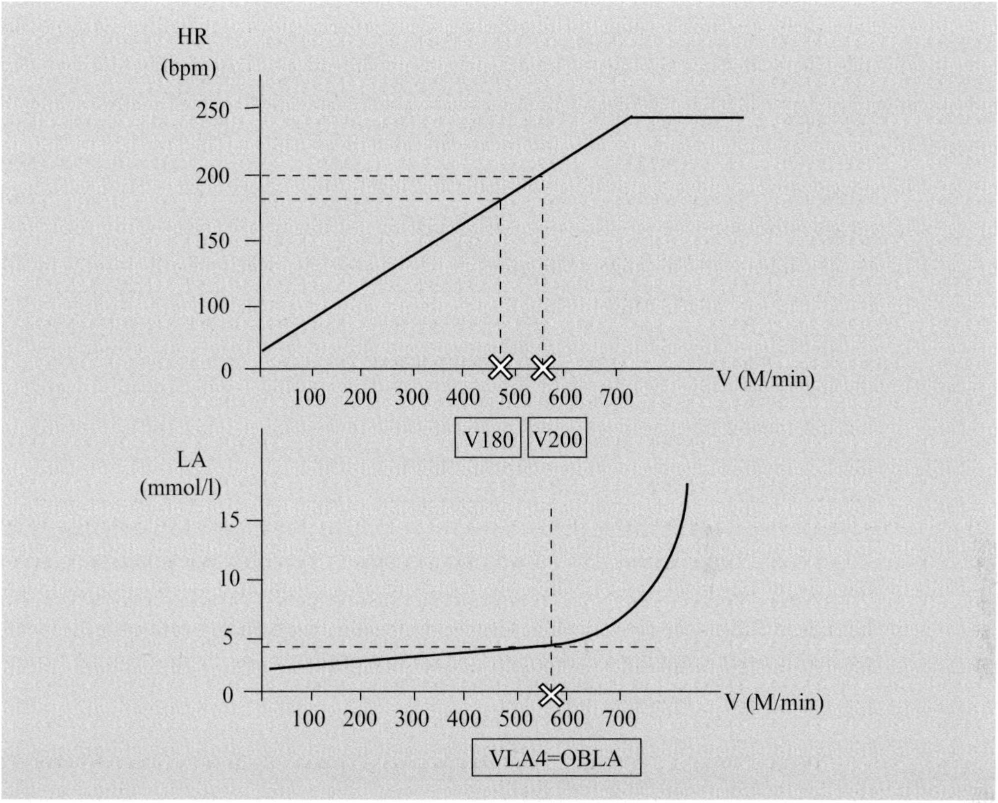

Figure 10. Heart rate (HR) and blood lactate (LA) vs speed. The dashed lines show how to evaluate V200 and VLA4 (see text for explanation).

Continuous **examination of the nasopharynx and larynx** during high-speed treadmill exercise is surely one of the major indications for treadmill tests. It offers the opportunity to see the dynamic phenomenon occurring at this level when soft tissues are submitted to high transmural pressures. Ideally, the test should be strenuous, but with saddle horses, it is sometimes impossible to perform very intense or exhausting exercise, or to recreate sufficient poll flexion similar to that imposed to the horse during riding.

It has been suggested that **arterial blood gas** measurements during exercise may contribute to establishing clinical diagnosis. The interpretation of the data of a single isolated tests is however problematic, as (1) hypoxemia and hypercapnia are known to occur in all athletic horses running at 60% or more of their VO_{2max} (Bayly, 1983); (2) hypoxemia and hypercapnia are more pronounced in well trained animals and in horses with high VO_{2max} (Art and Lekeux, 1993); (3) hypoxemia and hypercapnia are more pronounced in animals suffering from respiratory

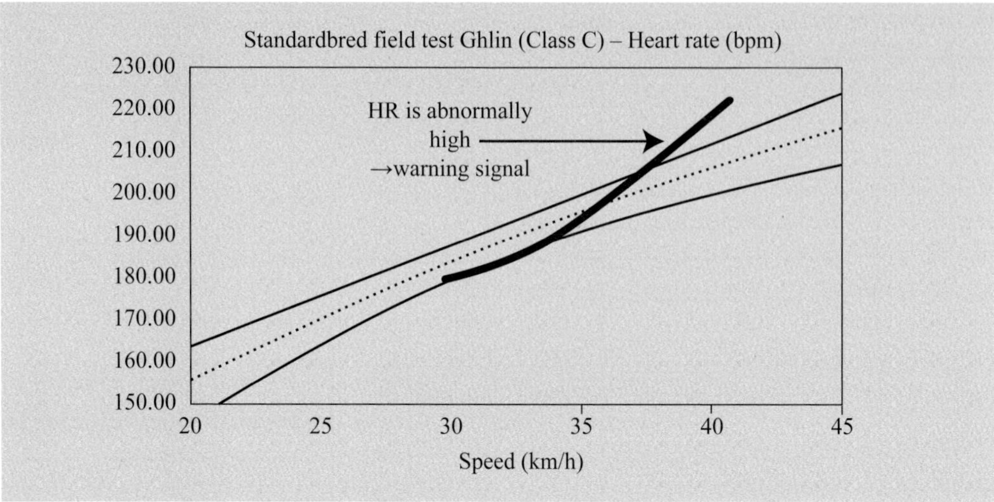

Figure 11. Heart rate reported as a function of speed in a standardbred racehorse suffering from exercise intolerance. The horse was within the norm during the first steps of the standardized test performed on the track, but had an abnormally high heart rate during the last step. This indicated the presence of a problem but did not give any diagnosis. Further examination performed on a treadmill revealed a dorsal displacement of the soft palate (Van Erck et al.*, 2006).*

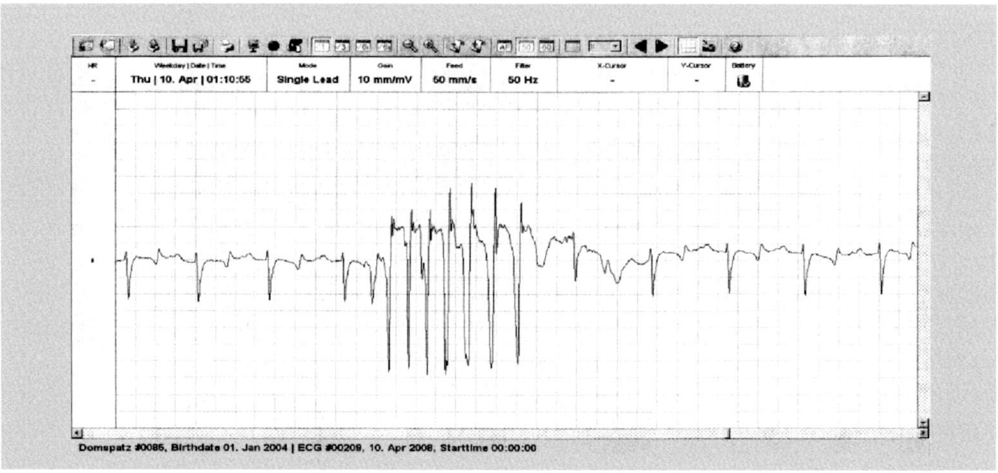

Figure 12. ECG from an international show jumping horse suffering from collapse syndrome during exercise. Salves of premature ventricular complexes were observed during the recovery phase.

diseases (Art *et al.*, 1998; Couetil and Denicola, 1999); (4) the data are only available for racing horses and not for saddle horses. Therefore, in the author's opinion, arterial blood gas measurements are justified only when performed by coupled and well standardized tests separated by a period sufficiently short to avoid training effects (eg before and after a surgical or medical treatments), or if associated with VO_{2max} measurements (with all the technical complexity inherent to such measurements).

Some equine sports physiologists advocate the measurement of the **oxygen consumption** (VO_2) especially during maximal exercise, to evaluate maximal aerobic power (Evans, 2007). This is considered as the gold standard in human sports medicine. Without doubt, the measurement of VO_{2max} is essential in research protocols, but to the authors' opinion, the technology is nowadays inapplicable in practice for numerous reasons. Firstly, the equipment is really expensive and consequently few laboratories are equipped with such a material; secondly, it requires wearing a mask which could be a problem with some nervous horses (necessitating a long acclimatization period) and could interfere with the normal respiratory physiology (especially at high exercise intensity); thirdly, this measurement is only valuable when performed at maximal and then supra-maximal exercise (in order to have a plateau in VO_2), an intensity that could be difficult to reach even with race horses and impossible to reach with jumping and endurance horses (Figure 13).

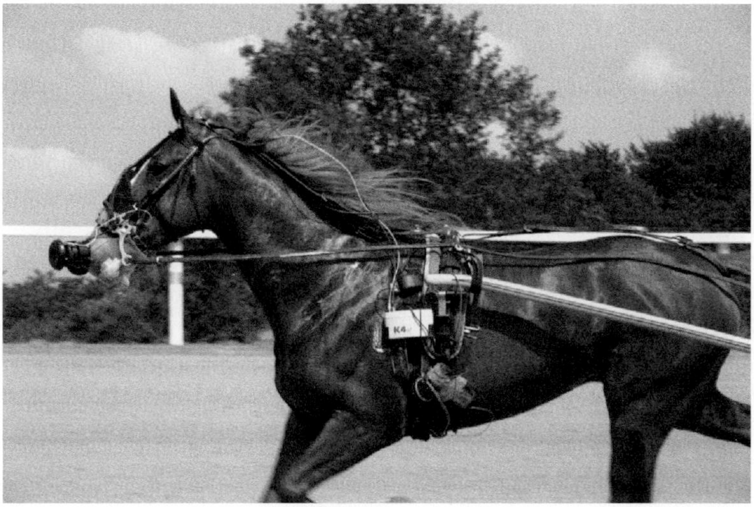

Figure 13. VO_2 measurement with a portable system on a Standardbred running on a racetrack during a research protocol aiming at studying the reliability of the system (Art et al.*, 2006) (Photo: Dr. R. Cedaro).*

Post-exercise

Immediately post-exercise (PE) echocardiography, ie stress echocardiography (0 to 2 minutes PE), cardiac recovery (during 15 minutes PE), muscular enzyme activity measurements such as CK (30-60 minutes PE), lower airway endoscopy (60 minutes PE) are complementary tests that provide further valuable information on the possible causes of exercise intolerance.

Lower airway endoscopy allows to examine the trachea and the bronchi and to assess the possible presence of mucus, mucopus or blood in the lower airway. Cytological examination of BAL is a sensitive and specific examination which assists in the diagnosis of lower airway disease, but yet does not give functional information on the existing problem. However, it is generally admitted that IAD and RAO are frequently in relation with exercise intolerance at least in racehorses.

Exercise tests: are they useful? Field or treadmill?

Diagnosis of the causes of exercise intolerance should never be based on a single measurement but integrated with the history, the clinical examination, and ancillary tests performed. The exercise test is one of these ancillary tests.

One of the biggest problems of the exercise tests is the fact that they may be difficult to interpret when performed once in the life of the horse, unless specific reference values are available for horses of similar age, training and level of competition, which is to this day the case only for standardbred horses (Couroucé 1999; Van Erck *et al.*, 2006) (Figure 14). Usually, a horse is referred for exercise testing only when it does not perform as expected by its trainer or owner. Ideally, exercise tests should be repeated at regular intervals in order to have the individual norms for a given horse. In this case, early changes in performance and problems could be detected more precociously. Moreover, as mentioned above, measurements such as VLA4 and V200 do not indicate specifically which particular system is deficient in the oxygen chain: they represent an objective warning signal that should encourage the practitioner to make further investigations.

The number of exercise protocols used probably reflects the number of laboratories that perform exercise tests. Fortunately, it is not important for an exercise test to be exactly the same in every laboratory or practice. But clearly, the tests should be standardized within a given practice. The exercise protocol may be adapted to the final aim of the test. Usually, to determine VLA4 and V200, a stepwise incremental test is used, while to induce UA dynamic obstruction, a test to exhaustion is preferred. While there seems to be a relative unanimity for the protocols to be used with Standardbreds (Couroucé, 1999) (Figure 15) and

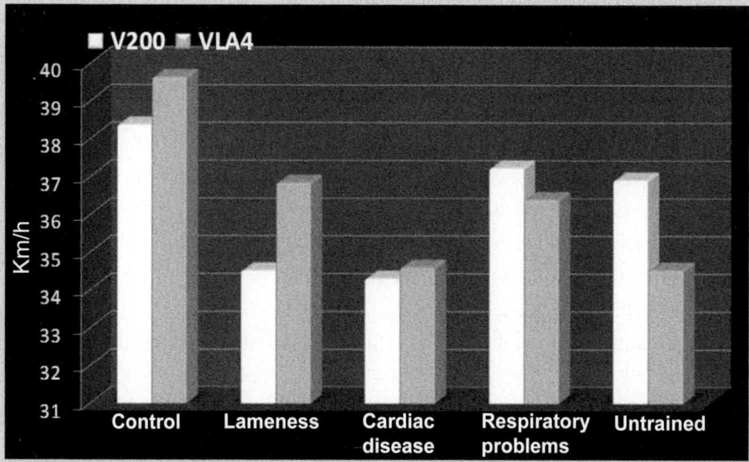

Figure 14. VLA4 and V200 measured in standardbred racehorses referred to the Equine Sports Medicine Center of Liege for exercise intolerance. Both parameters are decreased by the problems that have been diagnosed by further ancillary examinations (Van Erck et al.*, 2006).*

Categories	**A**	**B**	**C**
Warm-up (3500m)	3 laps at **20 km/h** (10 minutes)		
Step 1 (1500m)	**28 km/h** (7.8 m/s)	**29 km/h** (8.1 m/s)	**30 km/h** (8.3 m/s)
Step 2 (1500m)	**32 km/h** (8.9 m/s)	**33 km/h** (9.2 m/s)	**35 km/h** (9.7 m/s)
Step 3 (1500m)	**35 km/h** (9.7 m/s)	**38 km/h** (10.5 m/s)	**42 km/h** (11.7 m/s)
Active recovery (1000m)	1 lap at **20 km/h**		

Figure 15. Example of the standardized test for standardbred racehorses on the track used by the Equine Sports Medicine in Liege. Categories referred to the age and previous performances (Van Erck et al.*, 2006).*

Thoroughbreds, description of protocols for endurance, jumping and 3-day event horses are rare or not at all available. These horses have nevertheless different physiological, biomechanical and psychological specificities. For example, on the one hand, it is impossible to ask a near-maximal exercise test to a jumping or endurance horse and on the other hand, endurance horses are sometimes so well trained that they are unable to reach VLA4 or V200 on the treadmill. These horses should receive more attention from the scientific community, taking into account that they represent a non negligible part of many veterinary and laboratory practices.

Exercise tests may be performed for several purposes:
1. assessment of intrinsic athletic capacity;
2. assessment of fitness;
3. global examination of a poor performer without any evidence of abnormalities at rest;
4. confirmation during exercise that a problem identified or suspected on the basis of resting examination is a relevant cause of exercise intolerance.

From goal 1 to goal 4, the clinical reliability becomes better and the interpretation of the exercise test easier. Indeed, goal 1 remains very difficult to achieve outside real competitive circumstances. Goal 2 could be adequately reached if only regular tests were performed in the same horse and initial acquired data served as reference to assess progress during the training period. For goal 3, exercise tests are useful to indicate that the oxygen chain is somewhere disrupted or to demonstrate occurrence of pain or lameness. They may help to identify and/or prioritize causes of poor performance but may unfortunately be sometimes unconclusive. Surely, for goal 4, exercise tests are fully justified and useful, especially to elicit a problem occurring only at high level of exertion. E.g. exercise endoscopy helps to identify the origin of a respiratory noise and its functional significance, continuous ECG confirms the occurrence or disappearance of cardiac arrhythmia, and so on…

> A unique exercise test may be useful to examine a horse suffering from exercise intolerance, when a cause is suspected or even identified and need to be confirmed. Its use for the examination of a poor performer may be useful to identify and prioritize problems elicited by examination under exercise conditions but may be sometimes disappointing. The use of exercise tests for fitness assessment implies regular repetition of standardized tests to be easily interpretable.

Field or treadmill? Both locations have advantages and disadvantages (Sloet van Oldruitenborgh-Oosterbaan and Clayton, 1999).

Treadmill test has several advantages: standardization of exercise and environmental condition, easier use of equipments that enable measurements, namely to make exercise endoscopy, easy access to horse for cardio-respiratory measurements and blood sampling. It can be more stressful, especially for some individuals. Acclimatization to the treadmill is therefore recommended, though it makes the examination lengthier and more cumbersome.

Field exercise tests offer a more limited number of measurements to be done. It mimics the real work conditions and is therefore valuable to observe the behavior and gaits of the horse during its usual work; it is much less stressing for the horse and for the owner. Exercise is more difficult to standardize and to repeat in comparable conditions. The adaptation of new techniques for field measurements will certainly be a progress in the near future.

What is the future of sports medicine? New diagnostic tools for the future

1982: First International Congress of Equine Exercise Physiology: 'Exercise tests should allow for detecting causes of reduced performance and will be essential, in the future, in the evaluation of therapeutics required to restore or improve exercise tolerance'. Thomas & Fregin (Fregin and Thomas, 1982).

12 years later: 'Much of the basic knowledge of the physiology and biochemistry of equine exercise is now known. However, a great deal of the available information is purely descriptive, and therefore, considerable future research is required before specific recommendations can be made about optimal training methods or selection for performance'. Reuben Rose (Rose and Hodgson, 1994).

22 years later: 'More effort is needed to adapt new technologies, and, refine approaches to design field exercise tests and development of simple and user-friendly techniques for exercise studies of horses would therefore be a major advance … '. David Evans (Evans, 2004).

For a quarter of century, there has been a fantastic increase in our basic knowledge in equine exercise physiology and biochemistry. Nevertheless, it is obvious that the practical application, in the field, of these scientific advance progresses much more slowly than expected. The question is now why?

As already discussed, the diagnosis for poor performance and exercise intolerance would be facilitated if owners accepted a regular medical follow-up with possibly exercise tests. But they are reluctant to do so, and nowadays, they tend to consult only when the horse is a genuine poor performer or suffers from exercise intolerance. Why? Could it be that we, veterinarians and scientists, have been unable to demonstrate them the benefit of regular medico-sportive follow-up. Could it be the scientists were unable to fit the expectations of the horse's owners? Perhaps the latter find the methods used too heavy for them and too invasive for their horse?

How can we help the trainers and the owners to select high quality horses, to use their genetic potential with adequate training and management, and above all, to detect the potential problems when there are still subclinical? With simple and fast tests that are not too expensive and restricting?

We should focus:

- on exercise tests that may be also performed on jumping and endurance horses, without necessitating to conduct them up to exhaustion
- on pulmonary function tests that enable fast, non invasive, accurate and sensitive assessments of upper and lower airways;
- on the development of equipments allowing thorough examination on race track: telemetric endoscope is an example

Other solutions could be found in the future by the development of genomics, transcriptomics and proteomics. These emergent sciences in equine medicine could play a major role and offer a new way, simple and non invasive to identify factors involved in the occurrence of poor performance or exercise intolerance, biological samples (blood, BAL, ...) (Figure 16).

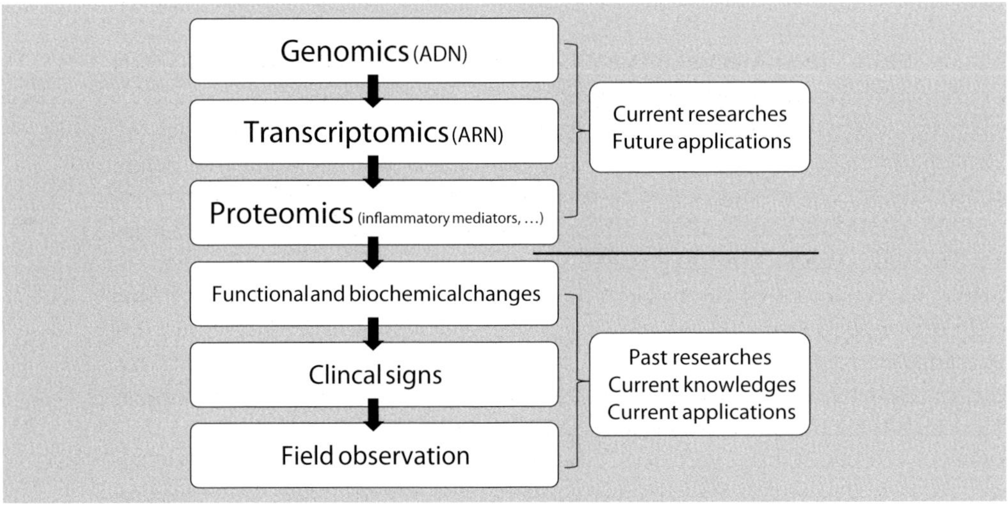

Figure 16. The way for the future: genomics, transcriptomics and proteomics.

References

Art, T. and P. Lekeux, 1993. Training-induced modifications in cardiorespiratory and ventilatory measurements in Thoroughbred horses. Equine Vet. J., 25: 532-536.

Art, T., D.H. Duvivier, D. Votion, N. Anciaux, S. Vandenput, W.M. Bayly and P. Lekeux, 1998. Does an acute COPD crisis modify the cardiorespiratory and ventilatory adjustments to exercise in horses? J. Appl. Physiol., 84: 845-852.

Art, T., D.H. Duvivier, E. Van Erck, B. De moffarts, D. Votion, D. Bedoret, J.P. Lejeune, P. Lekeux and D. Serteyn, 2006. Validation of a portable equine metabolic measurement system. Equine Vet. J., Suppl. 36: 557-561.

Bayly, W.M., B.D. Grant, R.G. Breeze and J.W. Kramer, 1983. The effects of maximal exercise on acid base balance and arterial blood gas tensions in Thoroughbred horses. In: D.H. Snow, S.G.B. Persson and R.J. Rose (Eds.) Equine Exercise Physiology, Granta Editions, Cambridge, pp 400-407.

Couëtil, L.L. and D.B. Denicola, 1999. Blood gas, plasma lactate and bronchoalveolar lavage cytology analyses in racehorses with respiratory disease. Equine Vet. J., Suppl. 30: 77-82.

Courouçé, A., 1999. Field exercise testing for assessing fitness in French Standardbred trotters. Vet. J., 157: 112-122.

Eaton, M.D., D.L. Evans, D.R. Hodgson and R.J. Rose, 1995. Assessment of anaerobic capacity using maximal accumulated oxygen deficit in fit Thoroughbreds. Equine Vet. J., Suppl. 18: 29-32.

Evans, D.L., 2004. Exercise testing in the field. In: K.W. Hinchcliffe, A.J. Kaneps and R.J. Geor (Eds.) Equine Sports Medicine and Surgery, W.B. Saunders, London, pp 19-31.

Evans, D.L., 2007. Physiology of equine performance and associated tests of function. Equine Vet. J., 39: 373-383.

Fregin, G.F. and D.P. Thomas, 1983. Cardiovascular Response to exercise in the horse: a review. In: D.H. Snow, S.G.B. Persson and R.J. Rose (Eds), Equine Exercise Physiology, Granta Editions, Cambridge, pp 400-407.

Martin, B.B. Jr, V.B. Reef, E.J. Parente and A.D. Sage, 2000. Causes of poor performance of horses during training, racing, or showing: 348 cases (1992-1996). J. Am. Vet. Med. Assoc., 216: 554-558.

Morris, E.A. and H.J. Seeherman, 1991. Clinical evaluation of poor performance in the racehorse: the results of 275 evaluations. Equine Vet. J., 23: 169-174.

Rose, R.J. and D.R. Hodgson, 1994. Clinical exercise testing. In: D.R. Hodgson and R.J. Rose (Eds.) The Athletic Horse: Principles and Practice of Equine Sports Medicine, W.B. Saunders Company, Philadelphia, pp. 245-257.

Sloet van Oldruitenborgh-Oosterbaan, M.M. and H.M. Clayton, 1999. Advantages and disadvantages of track vs treadmill tests. Equine Vet. JSuppl., 30: 645-647.

Van Erck, E., V. Jakesova, P. Lekeux and T. Art, 2006. Field evaluation of poor performance in Standardbred trotters. Pferdeheilkunde, 5: 625-631.

The gastrointestinal tract of performance horses: medical, nutritional and surgical considerations

Andy E. Durham[1] and Nathaniel A. White[2]
[1]The Liphook Equine Hospital, Forest Mere, Liphook, Hampshire, GU30 7EH, United Kingdom; andy@TheLEH.co.uk
[2]Marion duPont Scott Equine Medical Center, VMRCVM-Virginia Tech, Leesburg, Virginia 20177, USA; nawhite2@vt.edu

The equine digestive tract evolved anatomically and physiologically in an animal that led a relatively sedentary lifestyle continually browsing for fibre-rich and low-starch food (Houpt, 1990). Evolutionary survival pressures in a predated species inevitably led to a high capacity for sudden and high intensity exercise in response to perceived threats. Presumably such extreme exertion was relatively infrequent in the life of the ancestral feral equid as the dietary energy derived from available nutrient sources (grasses, rushes, sedges and perhaps occasional cereals) would probably be inadequate for daily high intensity or prolonged exercise. In a contrasting lifestyle, to facilitate and enhance performance of their intended sport, the almost daily exertional demands of the modern elite domesticated equid require a considerably increased quality and quantity of feed intake and also different feeding patterns and ingestive behaviours in comparison to the evolved physiologic template.

The National Research Council committee on nutrient requirements of horses recently stated that '*The goal of feeding management is to efficiently supply dietary ingredients in amounts that will meet the horse's nutrient needs, while still retaining the horse's normal feeding behaviour*' (National Research Council (NRC), 2007b). If '*normal feeding behaviour*' is taken to mean that to which horses have become adapted over 54 million years of evolution prior to their recent domestication, then this appears to be unachievable within the inevitable constraints of modern competition horse dietary management with possible adverse consequences on their gastrointestinal (GI) health. Increased exertional activity *per se* may have additional undesirable consequences on the GI tract.

In accordance with this dietary and behavioural divergence of the modern equine athlete from its feral ancestors, several studies have suggested that competition horses are at increased risk of GI disease (Archer and Proudman, 2006; Durham, 2007). Certain breeds such as the Thoroughbred and Arabian, developed for athletic pursuits, have been found to have inherently increased risk of GI disease (Cohen *et al.*, 1995b, 1999; Cohen and Peloso, 1996; Reeves *et al.*, 1996; Tinker *et al.*, 1997; Traub-Dargatz *et al.*, 2001). Eventing, race-training and showing activities have been found to be associated with more than double the risk of colic compared to non-competing horses (Kaneene *et al.*, 1997; Tinker *et al.*, 1997). However, other large epidemiologic studies have found no association between use of horse and colic risk (Traub-Dargatz *et al.*, 2001) and have even suggested that racehorses may have a lower colic risk than less physically active horses (Kaneene *et al.*, 1997; Cohen *et al.*, 1995b). Dehydration and loss of electrolytes from extended periods of exercise and transport have been associated with GI disturbances leading to colic, although only a few studies have established a significant association (Foreman, 1998; McCutcheon and Geor, 1998; Hillyer *et al.*, 2002). Prevalence studies of gastric ulcers reveal a strong association with exertional activities such as racing in Thoroughbreds and Standardbreds (Hammond *et al.*, 1986; Vatistas *et al.*, 1994; Rabuffo *et al.*, 2002; Dionne *et al.*, 2003; Bell *et al.*, 2007a), endurance races (Nieto *et al.*, 2004) western performance events (Bertone, 2000) and showing (McClure *et al.*, 1999).

This review considers the interactions between the equine GI tract and performance primarily in terms of dietary and exertional effects on GI health and also evidence linking these effects to performance. Although certain aspects of nutrition are considered, the reader is referred elsewhere within these proceedings for more specific discussion of nutrition and performance.

Dietary overview in the competition horse

Horses participating in different competitive pursuits frequently have markedly different dietary management and therefore subsequently differing health implications of the diets and the dietary interactions with training and competitive exertion. Diet quality may vary from the relatively high forage, low cereal diet of the endurance horse to the low forage, high cereal diet of the flat-racing Thoroughbred with intermediate gradations of dietary quality in other performance disciplines (Bishop, 2005; Geor and Harris, 2005; Richards *et al.*, 2006). Access to grazing varies considerably with generally greater access allowed for the endurance horse than the race horse (Geor and Harris, 2005; Bell *et al.*, 2007a). Fat-supplemented diets have become widely recommended, especially in endurance disciplines, in order to increase non-starch derived dietary energy with suggested relative benefits to GI health (Geor and Harris, 2005). Forage feeding immediately prior to training or racing in Thoroughbreds tends to be limited or absent resulting in exertion with a relatively empty stomach and colon, the former containing primarily gastric fluid and cereal. As forage intake will usually be accompanied by 3 to 4 times its weight in water intake (NRC, 2007a), the primary aim of forage restriction in racing Thoroughbreds is to reduce body mass and energy expenditure during exercise (Rice *et al.*, 2001; Ellis *et al.*, 2002). Horses fed 100% forage vs. hay plus concentrate have more weight and more heat production suggesting inefficiency in horses exercising on forage only diets (Kronfeld *et al.*, 1994; Kronfeld, 1996). Feeding grain immediately prior to exercise decreases free fatty acid availability and increased glucose disappearance during exercise. Feeding hay with grain or free choice the night before exercise decreased plasma volume and increased lactate and heart rate during exercise on a high-speed treadmill. Feeding only forage did not adversely affect performance but large amounts just prior to exercise could affect performance (Pagan and Harris, 1999). In contrast to racing Thoroughbreds, endurance horses are likely to have a GI tract filled with forage-based digesta at the time of competition, a status more similar to the likely evolutionary adaptation of the equine GI tract and providing an effective reservoir of nutrients, electrolytes and water. Fat adaptation further decreases heat production thereby reducing body temperature and needed daily water intake.

Dietary influences on gastric ulceration

Gastric ulceration is a disease of high prevalence in performance horses (Bell *et al.*, 2007b) and low-forage, high cereal diets have long been recognised in association with increased prevalence of gastric ulcers in racehorses (Hammond *et al.*, 1986). The upper squamous mucosa and lower glandular mucosa of the equine stomach have markedly different properties relevant to the interaction of diet and exercise with gastric disease (Merritt, 1999). Consistent with evolutionary development as a 'continual browser' or 'trickle-feeder', the equine stomach secretes hydrochloric acid (HCl) almost continually leading to normal prolonged exposure of glandular mucosa to acid (Campbell-Thompson and Merritt, 1990; Murray, 1997). Unsurprisingly development of a strong antacid defence can be demonstrated in this ventral area of the stomach consisting of prostaglandin-dependent secretion of bicarbonate-rich mucus, good mucosal blood flow (to remove any penetrating protons and maintain potential for a high metabolic rate) and rapid restitution following erosion or ulceration of the epithelium (Murray, 1999). Observations of the pH and gross appearance of fibrous ingesta within the forage-fed equine stomach suggest that the gastric squamous mucosa did not evolve in frequent contact with low pH gastric fluid and has not suffered strong evolutionary pressure to develop robust antacid defence unlike its subjacent neighbour (Ethell *et al.*, 2000). The stomach content of a horse fed forage/grass *ad libitum* tends to be a solid but stratified mass of increasing pH from highly acidic ventrally adjacent to the acid-secreting glandular mucosa, to neutral or alkaline pH at the most dorsal aspect of the mass of ingesta exposed to salivary bicarbonate entering the cardia within the squamous mucosal area (Figure 1). Forage filling the stomach serves to limit mixing and movement of acidic fluid within the stomach and also incurs a considerably increased secretion of salivary buffer than does a cereal diet (Meyer *et al.*, 1985). High-cereal (and low-forage) consumption may promote fluidity, mixing and agitation of gastric contents by reducing intragastric dry matter (Figure 2) and therefore increase the potential for contact of the poorly defended squamous mucosa with low pH gastric fluid.

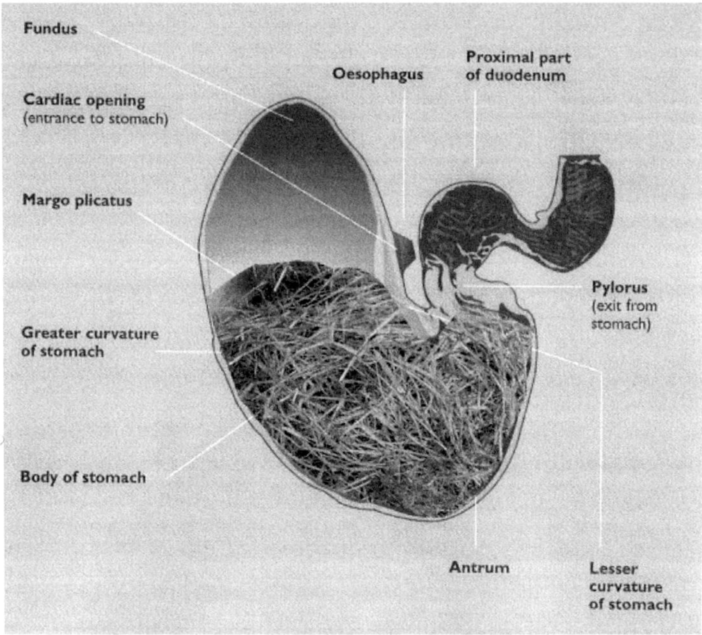

Figure 1. Diagramatic representation of the normal ad lib *forage-fed equine stomach with solid, pH-stratified forage content (Murray and Grodinsky, 1989; Merritt, 2003).*

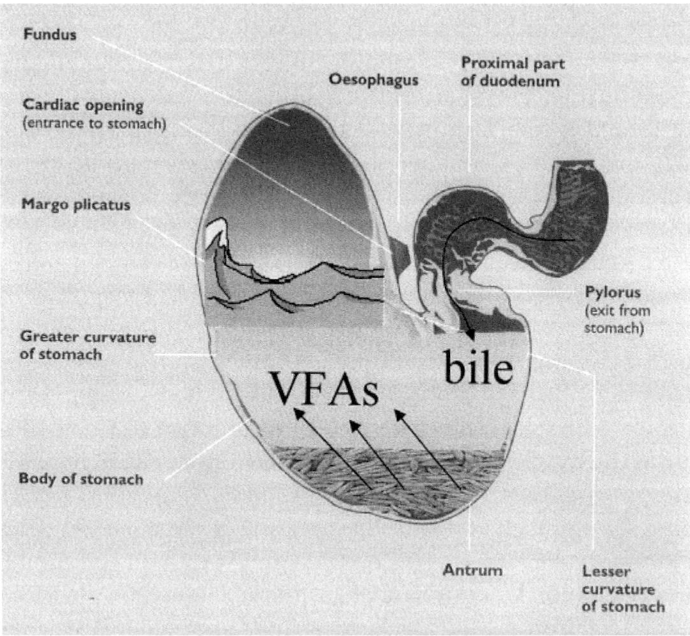

Figure 2. Diagrammatic representation of the high-cereal, low-forage fed equine stomach with freely moving and mixing acidic liquid content fortified with VFAs and bile (Argenzio, 1999).

Additionally high cereal diets may stimulate a more prolonged gastrin secretory response (Smyth *et al.*, 1989; Sandin *et al.*, 1998) further increasing the corrosive properties of gastric fluid.

The harmful effect of HCl may be compounded by the presence of volatile fatty acids (VFAs) in the gastric fluid. VFAs such as acetic, propionic, butyric, valeric and isovaleric acids arise from fermentation of food (especially starches) within the stomach. Furthermore, high-starch meals tend to reduce gastric emptying rates (Metayer *et al.*, 2004) and therefore further promote fermentative production of VFAs. The pKa of most VFAs found in the equine stomach is between 4 and 5 and thus they will be primarily in their non-ionised form in low pH gastric fluid. Diffusion of VFAs across squamous mucosal cell membranes is facilitated by their non-ionised, hydrophobic status and subsequent dissociation of their hydrogen ion within the nearly neutral pH of the cytosol may cause harmful intracellular acidification and cell death (Nadeau *et al.*, 2003a,b; Andrews *et al.*, 2006). Alfalfa feeding may offer a protective effect by buffering gastric fluid and reducing mucosal uptake of VFAs in comparison to grass hays (Nadeau *et al.*, 2000; Lybbert *et al.*, 2007).

Consistent with an evolutionary adaptation to continual feed intake, feed deprivation and intermittent feeding programmes have been shown to be an effective means of squamous mucosal ulcerogenesis in experimental studies in horses (Murray and Eichorn 1996). When the equine stomach is continually filled with high-fibre material there are beneficial consequences beyond the buffering and stabilisation effect of the solid mass of fibrous ingesta described above. Additionally, reflux and dispersal of pancreatic and biliary secretions within the stomach is physically limited in comparison to a forage-restricted diet when the stomach is largely devoid of solidly structured matter. As the equine pylorus offers little resistance to retrograde flow, frequent boluses of pancreatic and biliary secretion will enter the stomach and mix freely in an empty or fluid-filled stomach (Figure 2). Although there may be significant buffering of gastric acid by pancreatic bicarbonate (Merritt 1999), the presence of bile acids within gastric fluid may be harmful to the mucosa and this is consistent with the relatively high prevalence of ulcers in the pyloric area in competition horses (Murray *et al.*, 2001; Begg and O'Sullivan, 2003; Bell *et al.*, 2007a). As described above for VFAs, bile acids in their non-ionised form within the low pH gastric fluid may diffuse into mucosal cells leading to cell death and necrosis (Argenzio, 1999; Berschneider *et al.*, 1999; Murray, 1999) although this is not a theory supported by all studies (Widenhouse *et al.*, 2002). Bile acids might further disrupt the protective phospholipid barrier covering the squamous mucosal surface (Geor, 2000). Dietary oils have been proposed as a means of defending against gastric ulceration. Possible beneficial mechanisms of action might include provision of substrate for prostaglandin synthesis (likely to primarily aid gastric *glandular* mucosal defence) or possibly by binding free bile acids within the gastric fluid. However, studies have not consistently found dietary oils to reduce gastric ulcers in horses (Cargile *et al.*, 2004; Frank *et al.*, 2005).

Hypertonic electrolyte solutions and pastes are sometimes administered to horses with the intention of improving performance, hydration and electrolyte status in endurance competitions and this has also been reported as a more surreptitious practice in Thoroughbred and Standardbred racing (Rose and Lloyd, 1992; Auer *et al.*, 1993; Nyman *et al.*, 1996). This treatment may be significantly harmful to the gastric squamous mucosa and has been associated with significant squamous ulcerogenesis (Holbrook *et al.*, 2005).

Dietary influences on intestinal digestion and fermentation

The horse's GI tract has evolved to function for a grazing animal that has frequent periods of forage intake interspersed with periods of rest and movement to new food sources. The small intestine serves for energy absorption including sugars, starch, protein and fat. The large intestine or hindgut has adapted for microbial digestion of starch and fibre. Because of the likely inefficient digestion of starch in the horse's small intestine, when grain is fed rapidly fermentable starch is passed into the large intestine. Rapid fermentation of starch in the large intestine (caecum and large colon) alters volatile fatty acid ratios (increased proprionate and decreased acetate) and increases lactate production (Geor and Harris, 2007). A decrease in butyrate transport in the mucosa is altered as well as the increased production of vasoactive substances such as monoamines, endotoxin and exotoxins (Bailey *et al.* 2002, 2003; Geor and Harris, 2007). The decreased intake of slow fermenting carbohydrates (cellulose, hemicellulose, ligno-cellulose) decreases the water content in the large colon potentially affecting energy production (decreased acetate), water reserve in the colon and weight. Less fibre with increased starch in the diet decreases water in the colon ingesta and increases gas production (Lopes *et al.*, 2004).

Alterations in diet to provide needed energy for performance is associated with an increased risk of colic due to higher levels of cereal or concentrate feeding (Tinker *et al.*, 1997, Hudson *et al.*, 2001; Cohen *et al.*, 2006). Incomplete pre-caecal digestion of starch has long been recognised for its potential adverse effect on large bowel health and function (Goodson *et al.*, 1988; Clarke *et al.*, 1990; de Fombelle *et al.*, 2001; Drogoul *et al.*, 2001; Julliand *et al.*, 2001; Hussein *et al.*, 2004; Lopes *et al.*, 2004) and levels as low as 1g starch per kg bodyweight per meal (eg. 1 kg concentrate feed for a Thoroughbred) could overwhelm the limited digestive capacity of the equine small intestine (Potter *et al.*, 1992) especially if starch sources of low digestibility are fed (Cuddeford, 2000; Hintz, 2000; Hussein *et al.*, 2004). Richards *et al.* (2006) reported a mean grain intake of 7.3 kg/day (range 3.8-13.2 kg/day) for racing Thoroughbreds in Australia and 27% of horses studied had faecal pH <6.2 that is likely to be associated with an adverse colonic environment for mucosal barrier function and survival of fibre-fermenting bacterial species. The digestibility of fibre, the nutrients for which the equine digestive tract is apparently best adapted, is significantly reduced by cereal feeding and this effect is further exacerbated by exercise (Pagan *et al.*, 1998). The adaptation to fat digestibility appears to be a way to avoid high starch intake while maintaining adequate energy intake and glucose metabolism during exercise (Kronfeld, 1996; Treiber *et al.*, 2006). To date there does not appear to be increased risk of colic associated with fat in the form of vegetable oils although some studies have found significantly reduced cellulolytic capacity of the equine hindgut with high fat diets (Jansen *et al.*, 2002), and the full effect of fat added to the diet in relation to performance is not yet known (Zeyner *et al.*, 2002).

General relationship between exercise and the GI tract

Exercise in humans and horses is associated with increases in several hormones that may affect GI secretion, motility, perfusion, absorption and permeability including catecholamines, cholecystokinin, cortisol, dopamine, endorphins, gastrin, glucagon, glucagon-like peptide 1, motilin, neurokinin A, pancreastatin, pancreatic polypeptide, peptide histidine isoleucine, peptide YY, prostaglandins, secretin, somatostatin, and vasoactive intestinal polypeptide (Demers *et al.*, 1981; Hall *et al.*, 1982; Woie *et al.*, 1986; Brouns and Beckers, 1993; O'Connor *et al.*, 1995; Nagata *et al.*, 1999). Exercise may be beneficial or harmful to GI structure and function depending on the nature and intensity of the exercise and the status of the GI tract at the time of exertion. In general mild to moderate aerobic exercise has been found to have significant beneficial effects on human GI function whereas intense or prolonged endurance exercise is frequently harmful (Moses, 1990; Brouns and Beckers, 1993; Peters *et al.*, 2001; Simrén 2002; Bi and Triadafilopoulos, 2003). Physical activity in humans has been found to have a marked beneficial effect on the risk of colon cancer (Thune and Furberg, 2001) and also on other intestinal complaints such as diverticular disease (Aldoori *et al.*, 1995), constipation (de Schryver *et al.*, 2005) and inflammatory bowel disease (Klein *et al.*, 1998). In marked contrast however, public marathon races have been described as a '*preplanned mass casualty incident*' with acute GI disease being one of the most common medical complaints amongst human competitors (Sanchez *et al.*, 2006). Between 30 and 81% of human marathon runners describe unpleasant GI symptoms during a race (Sullivan and Wong, 1992; Lucas and Schroy, 1998; Gil *et al.*, 1998; Sanchez *et al.*, 2006) and this is exacerbated by associated dehydration and hypovolaemia (Rehrer *et al.*, 1990; Brouns and Beckers 1993). Between 8 and 85% of human distance runners have positive faecal occult blood after a race (Choi *et al.*, 2001; Sanchez *et al.*, 2006) and also faecal α_1 antitrypsin and lysozyme concentrations are increased following prolonged exercise in humans and dogs indicating mucosal inflammation and damage (Peters *et al.*, 2000a; Davis *et al.*, 2006). Voluntary exercise in rats is associated with caecal enlargement and beneficial effects on its bacterial and VFA content in comparison to sedentary controls (Matsumoto *et al.*, 2008). In contrast, intense exercise appears to be rapidly and significantly harmful to the structure and function of the murine intestine with mucosal necrosis, damage to muscular layers and inhibition of motility all being reported (de Lira *et al.*, 2008; Rosa *et al.*, 2008).

There are few studies of the effects of exercise on GI disease in horses although the majority appear to suggest a deleterious effect of exercise on GI health. As discussed above several, but not all, studies have found a higher incidence of colic in horses that were actively training and competing. Hillyer *et al.* (2001) found that the months of peak incidence of colic in racing Thoroughbreds (flat and National Hunt) coincided with the timing of peak exertional activity although whether this effect was directly associated with exercise or perhaps confounded by diet or other factors was not examined. In a multivariate analysis where confounding factors were controlled, Cohen *et al.* (1999) found that horses exercised at least once each week had a significantly increased risk of colic when compared with horses living at pasture (OR 1.6; 95% CI 1.2-2.2; P=0.003). Similarly training and competition is well recognised to be associated with development of gastric ulcers in horses (Hammond *et al.*, 1986; Vatistas *et al.*, 1999a; Hartmann *et al.*, 2003; McClure *et al.*, 2005; White *et al.*, 2007) although again confounding factors make it impossible to directly attribute this effect to exercise and reports of a high prevalence of gastric ulcers in sedentary grazing horses also casts doubt on this putative relationship (le Jeune *et al.*, 2006). In contrast, observations consistent with a possible beneficial effect of exercise on GI motility and impaction colic are published. Impaction colic has frequently been noted to follow a reduction in exercise (Love *et al.*, 1994; Dabareiner and White, 1995; Hillyer *et al.*, 2002; Cox *et al.*, 2007) although this relationship might be confounded by associated dietary changes or other factors such as pain from musculoskeletal injury (a possible cause of the reduction in exercise) or medication (eg nonsteroidal anti-inflammatory drugs (NSAIDs)). Several possible mechanisms by which exercise could influence GI health and function are discussed below.

Exercise and intestinal barrier function

In humans and horses there is a reduction in intestinal blood flow by as much as 80% in response to exercise with even greater exercise-related hypoperfusion of the equine pancreas and stomach having been measured (Manohar, 1986; Manohar *et al.*, 1995; Clausen, 1997). Increased blood viscosity and cellularity associated with exercise in horses may further compromise mucosal perfusion

(Geor *et al.*, 1994). Non-endocrine mechanisms such as the significantly increased intrabdominal pressure seen at the start of exertional activity (Lorenzo-Figueras and Merritt, 2002) might also adversely affect splanchnic perfusion. Reduced GI perfusion could lead to pain and/or compromise of the mucosal barrier (Pals *et al.*, 1997). Cortisol has been found to increase GI permeability and the increased cortisol secretion found especially during endurance exercise (Nagata *et al.*, 1999) could further exacerbate the effects of reduced perfusion on mucosal integrity and subsequently allow access of endotoxin and other noxious substances into the peripheral circulation (Fink *et al.*, 1991). NSAID use at the time of a competitive race is discouraged in human athletes owing to the potential additive deleterious effect of these drugs on intestinal permeability (Smetanka *et al.*, 1999; Lambert *et al.*, 2007). In humans and horses plasma endotoxin levels increase significantly after intense or prolonged exercise (Cannon and Kluger, 1983; Baker *et al.*, 1988; Bosenberg *et al.*, 1988; Sakurada and Hales, 1998; Barton *et al.*, 2003) and intestinal permeability has been shown to increase with relatively modest exercise in dogs (Davis *et al.*, 2006). Plasma collected from humans after exercise caused pyrexia when transfused into rats, whereas pre-exercise plasma did not, indicating an exercise-induced accumulation of endogenous pyrogens (presumably endotoxin) in the circulation (Cannon and Kluger, 1983) and suggesting a role for intestinal-derived endotoxin in the hyperthermic response to intense exercise.

Exercise, intestinal motility and absorption

Studies of the effects of exercise on intestinal transit and absorption generally lack consensus. Generally mild intensity exercise appears to improve or have no effect on gastric emptying in humans although gastric emptying is significantly delayed by intense exercise in humans perhaps as a result of increased levels of catecholamines and endorphins (Neufer *et al.*, 1989; Rehrer *et al.*, 1990; Leiper *et al.*, 2005). Some human studies have found orocaecal transit time and colon motility are increased by exercise whereas others have not (Gisolfi, 2000; Peters *et al.*, 2001). Putative deleterious effects of exercise on intestinal absorption in humans are equivocal and the effects, if present, are probably not marked (Gisolfi, 2000; Lang *et al.*, 2006). Similarly, several studies have failed to find a marked effect of exercise on GI motility and absorption in horses and donkeys (Orton *et al.*, 1985b; Pearson and Merritt, 1991; Sosa Léon *et al.*, 1997; Pagan *et al.*, 1998). Equine studies have shown slightly increased dry matter intake *and* increased digestibility of the dry matter in association with light exercise consistent with slower intestinal transit (Olsson and Ruudvere, 1955; Orton *et al.*, 1985a, b). In a study using yearling horses, Orton *et al.* (1985b) found that trotting (12 km/h) for 1 hour/day prolonged the mean retention time of a marker of fluid digesta (^{51}Cr-EDTA) whereas a marker of particulate digesta (ruthenium-phenanthroline) was more rapidly eliminated in the faeces of the exercising horses. Overall digestibility was improved by light exercise and this was explained by the fluid phase containing the more digestible dietary elements. A further study by Pagan *et al.* (1998) examined the effect of more intense exercise on parameters of digestibility and intestinal transit in adult Thoroughbred geldings subject to a gradually increasing treadmill exercise programme culminating in speeds of 4-9 km/hr over 8 km at a 3° incline. In contrast to the study by Orton *et al.* (1985b), exercise resulted in a small but significant decrease in dry matter digestibility, largely because of decreased acid detergent fibre digestibility. However, exercise led to more rapid elimination of a particulate marker of digesta (Ytterbium chloride) in accordance with the previous study.

Electrolytes and water: effect on performance and colic

Dehydration and electrolyte imbalance are considered risks for colic as well as affecting performance (Foreman, 1998; Naylor *et al.*, 1993). Colic causes dehydration either by lack of intake or by 3rd space sequestration depending on the severity of the obstruction. Horses suffering from dehydration cannot perform optimally. The best examples are endurance horses or three-day event horses which suffer dehydration due to sweating particularly in hot weather. Continued sweating in the face of dehydration does not affect the amount of sweat produced thereby exacerbating dehydration if there is no fluid replacement. However, acclimation over time in hot environments decreases sweat rate (McCutcheon *et al.*, 1999). Though horses start to rehydrate after exercise with normal oral intake, full rehydration is not completed for 24-48 hours (Butudom *et al.*, 2003). The time required for full recovery without supplementation has not been reported and optimal performance is unlikely until hydration status has returned to normal.

Losses due to sweating during long distance exercise also causes sodium, potassium calcium and chloride depletion (Carlson and Mansmann, 1974; Rose *et al.*, 1980), though when supplementation occurred all electrolyte concentrations increased with an increased PCV (Hess *et al.*, 2005). Hypokalaemia and hypocalcaemia, which have been detected in dehydrated and exhausted horses, are associated with paralytic ileus. The resulting functional obstruction potentially creates more dehydration and electrolyte imbalance.

Synchronous diaphragmatic flutter, an indication of electrolyte imbalance (hypochloraemia, hypokalaemia and hypocalcaemia) during exercise, is associated with ileus or colic (Mansmann *et al.*, 1974; White, 1998). Hypocalcaemia and hypomagnesaemia have been recognized during colic requiring surgery and strangulating diseases and can be associated with cardiac dysrhythmias and ileus (Dart *et al.*, 1992; Garcia-Lopez *et al.*, 2001). Intravenous treatment with calcium borogluconate and or magnesium chloride is recommended. Correction is often immediate though magnesium may require oral supplementation for several days to replenish a deficiency.

Exercise, competition and gastric ulceration

Diet appears to have a significant influence on development of gastric ulcers in performance horses as discussed above. However, a study by Bell *et al.* (2007a), which found no protective effect of grazing on the development of gastric ulcers in racehorses, emphasised the likelihood of a direct association between other factors such as exercise with ulcerogenesis also. Gastritis is a well-recognised consequence of prolonged exercise in humans and dogs (Simons and Kennedy, 2004; Davis *et al.*, 2005, 2006) and has been mainly attributed to decreased GI perfusion, a key element of glandular mucosal defence (Murray, 1992a, 1999). Antacid therapy significantly reduces the incidence and severity of exercise-associated gastritis in humans and dogs suggesting acid-related factors in the aetiology (Choi *et al.*, 2006; Williamson *et al.*, 2007). Training significantly increases serum gastrin levels in response to feeding in horses (Furr *et al.*, 1994) and may be a contributor to exercise induced gastric acidity and ulceration. Gastric ulceration is common in exercising horses although gastric glandular mucosal ulcers (analogous to human and canine gastric lesions) are rare in comparison to squamous mucosal ulcers (Murray *et al.*, 1996, 2001) suggesting different aetiology of exercise-associated gastric disease in the horse versus the human and dog. Gastro-oesophageal reflux, a human condition more closely related to gastric squamous mucosal ulceration in horses, is also frequently associated with exercise in humans and has been attributed to the combination of increased intra-abdominal pressure and decreased intra-thoracic pressure at peak inhalation during exercise (Peters *et al.*, 2000b; Jozkow *et al.*, 2006). Lorenzo-Figueras and Merritt (2002) found the intragastric pressure to increase suddenly and markedly at the walk-trot transition in horses presumably due to external compression following increased tone of abdominal muscles. Furthermore, gastric fluid pH decreased to <4 during trotting and galloping and did not increase until the horse returned to walking. It was suggested that this effect would raise the intragastric fluid level and promote contact of low pH gastric fluid with the upper squamous mucosa although oesophageal reflux was not studied.

The inevitable physical agitation of abdominal viscera during exercise may well have adverse effects on the GI tract and the frequency of most GI symptoms in humans is almost twice as high during running than in less vibrational and concussive exercise such as cycling and swimming (Sullivan, 1987; Rehrer and Meijer, 1991; Peters *et al.*, 2000b). Rapid and forceful diaphragmatic movements during exercise might also contribute to GI disturbance. Equine gaits faster than a walk are all fairly concussive and could theoretically have many adverse consequences such as stretching, compression, bouncing and displacement of various viscera, mesentery and blood vessels and also significant abnormal agitation and disturbance of the normal movement of ingesta contained within. Jumping activities might be even more disruptive. Exercise-associated splashing of low pH gastric fluid may contribute to squamous mucosal ulceration in exercising horses. It is common for racehorses to be exercised when the stomach is relatively free of food content. This practice is partly based on the analogy that human athletes feel uncomfortable if running with a full stomach but it does inevitably promote agitation, movement and splashing of acidic fluid within the stomach during exercise especially if dietary management has promoted fluid gastric content (see above). Although human athletes suffer a high incidence of gastric symptoms during endurance exercise, the contact of low pH fluid with the equine squamous mucosa is likely to be even more poorly defended than that within the human stomach. Thus on the one hand we have a problem with exercising on a full stomach, and on the other we have a problem with exercising on an empty stomach. The premise that horses have probably not evolved to undergo frequent intense or prolonged endurance exercise, indicates that there may not necessarily be a satisfactory solution to this quandary although more consideration might be given to feeding long-fibre pre-exercise to encourage a more physically stable and pH-stratified gastric content (Murray and Grodinsky, 1989; Merritt, 2003).

Further experiences of the performance horse may contribute to gastric ulceration such as transport and stress (McClure *et al.*, 2005) and horses with a more nervous disposition have been found to be predisposed to ulceration (McClure *et al.*, 1999). However, theoretically stress and cortisol-mediated prostaglandin suppression would be more likely to affect gastric glandular defence and therefore promote glandular rather than squamous mucosal ulceration (Furr *et al.*, 1992; Murray, 1999). It may be the case that interruption of dietary patterns, alimentary secretions and even physical vibrational/agitational effects of transport might confound the proposed association between stress and squamous mucosal ulceration in adult horses (McClure *et al.*, 2005).

NSAIDs and GI disease

Given the frequency of orthopaedic injury and disease in performance horses, NSAIDs are probably the commonest prescribed medication in this group of animals (Kallings, 1993). NSAIDs antagonise prostaglandin-dependent mucosal defence and integrity of the GI tract (Wilson 1991) and NSAID therapy has been associated with protein losing enteropathy, gastric ulcers and right dorsal colitis in horses (Karcher *et al.*, 1990; Monreal *et al.*, 2004; Reed *et al.*, 2006).

NSAID-induced gastric ulceration occurs primarily, but not exclusively, in the prostaglandin-dependent gastric *glandular* mucosa (Monreal *et al.*, 2004), a relatively uncommonly ulcerated area in competition horses (Vatistas *et al.*, 1999b; Murray *et al.*, 2001; Begg and O'Sullivan, 2003; Nieto *et al.*, 2004). However, NSAIDs might also have a local direct adverse effect on mucosal surface protective phospholipids and cell membranes and therefore potentially contribute to gastric squamous mucosal ulcers in this way (Lichtenberger *et al.*, 2006). Whatever the exact mechanism of NSAID-induced gastric ulcers, there appears to be little evidence that NSAID therapy at commonly used doses is a significant cause of gastric ulceration in horses (Hammond *et al.*, 1986; Murray *et al.*, 1996; Vatistas *et al.*, 1999b; Rabuffo *et al.*, 2002; Reed *et al.*, 2006).

The health and function of the right dorsal colon appears especially NSAID-sensitive and right dorsal colitis is a well recognised, albeit uncommon, consequence of NSAID therapy in horses (Karcher *et al.*, 1990; Bueno *et al.*, 2000) and it has been suggested that young performance horses are especially predisposed (Cohen 2002). Right dorsal colitis is most commonly associated with excessive NSAID dosing but some cases occur with short term and appropriate dose regimens (Cohen *et al.*, 1995a). No difference in the right dorsal colonic mucosa was observed during experimental administration of phenylbutazone for 28 days (McConnico *et al.*, 2006), however, right dorsal colonic blood flow was significantly increased suggesting a systemic effect of chronic administration.

It is important to remember that NSAIDs may be a cause of protein losing enteropathy, hypoproteinaemia and weight loss in horses prior to development of obvious clinical signs of gastric or colonic disease (Reed *et al.*, 2006).

Relationship between the GI tract, training and performance

The putative association between GI disease and poor performance is generally ascribed in terms of anecdote and intuition rather than evidence and does not feature at all in 2 large reviews including 623 poor performance cases (Morris and Seeherman, 1991; Martin *et al.*, 2000). Traub-Dargatz *et al.* (2001) estimated that 2.2 days of use are lost per colic episode in horses although this is unlikely to have a major impact on training or competition unless occurring at key times.

In addition to the more familiar adaptations to physical training in the cardiopulmonary and musculoskeletal systems, adaptation of the GI tract may also be an important and beneficial component of training. Exercise-associated splanchnic hypoperfusion, loss of barrier function and endotoxaemia as discussed above may be an important cause of fatigue via effects on hyperthermia, hyperlactaemia and cardiac contractility (Cannon and Kluger, 1983; Abel, 1989; Williamson and Barton, 1996; Barton *et al.*, 2003). Ovine studies have suggested that improved heat tolerance associated with training results from reduced endotoxin absorption from the better perfused intestine of physically fit versus sedentary animals (Sakurada and Hales, 1998). Furthermore, actively competing humans and horses have high levels of anti-endotoxin antibodies suggesting chronic/repeated exposure to endotoxin and, possibly, greater tolerance of exercise-associated endotoxaemia and its putative adverse effects described above (Baker *et al.*, 1988; Bosenberg *et al.*, 1988); although a consistent correlation between level of physical fitness or performance and endotoxin antibodies has not been shown (Camus *et al.*, 1997; Barton *et al.*, 2003).

Although several studies have shown reduced gastric emptying in humans in response to intense exercise, trained endurance athletes were found to have faster gastric emptying rates than sedentary controls both at rest and during exercise suggesting gastric adaptation to exercise (Carrió *et al.*, 1989). However the suggested mechanism for this adaptation is enhanced gastric distension associated with a greater food intake by highly active human athletes. In an equine context the opposite effect might actually be the case when the volume of a concentrate-rich competition diet is compared with a high-forage, lower energy diet of more sedentary horses.

Gastric ulceration is the most frequently discussed GI disease of competition horses. Studies of gastric ulcers in adult horses have most frequently found signs such as weight loss, poor appetite, poor hair coat, colic and diarrhoea (Murray *et al.*, 1989; Murray, 1992b; Vatistas *et al.*, 1999b; Dionne *et al.*, 2003; Stämpfli and Oliver, 2006). Several publications describe decreased performance as a consequence of the disease (Murray, 1992b; Andrews and Nadeau, 1999; Equine Gastric Ulcer Council, 1999) despite an absence of good quality evidence existing to justify this widely accepted association. In a study of 202 Thoroughbreds in active race training, Vatistas *et al.* (1999b) compared the prevalence of gastric ulcers against the trainers' subjective assessments of performance (NB not all horses had previously trained or raced). Those horses performing 'at or above expectation' had a significantly lower prevalence of ulcers than those horses performing 'below expectations' (78% vs 94%, P=0.01). However, the severity or number of ulcers was not correlated with the degree of under-performance. Mitchell (2001) studied 134 hunter/jumper and dressage horses with a complaint of poor performance and other signs consistent with gastric ulcers and found gastric ulcers in 84 (63%) of them. Following treatment with omeprazole a '*noticeable improvement in performance within 5-7 days*' was frequently seen and '*trainers consistently related that treated horses were more willing to work*'. In a study of 80 racing Standardbreds, Jonsson and Egenvall (2006) found a higher prevalence of gastric ulcers in horses performing 'worse than expected' (66.7%) than in groups performing 'better than expected' (36.4%) or 'as expected' (31.1%). Although these data illustrated a significant association between trainers' expectations and prevalence of gastric ulceration, this only remained significant (P=0.002) in univariable analysis and may have been confounded by other factors. Furthermore, the prevalence of ulcers in horses performing 'better than expected' was greater than in those performing 'as expected'. Johnson *et al.* (2001) examined 565 horses with trainer complaints thought to be compatible with gastric ulceration and 506 (90%) were indeed confirmed to have gastric ulcers and were then treated with omeprazole. Performance in the 6 months preceding the trial was then compared with performance in the 6 months following treatment of the gastric ulcers. Before the trial 40% of horses finished races in the top 3 whereas this proportion increased to 46% after treatment for ulcers although statistical comparison of these findings was not described. Franklin *et al.* (2008) described 4 poorly performing Thoroughbred racehorses in which no abnormalities other than gastric ulceration were found. Performance judged by Raceform rating and earnings of each horse was improved following treatment with omeprazole.

There are many trainer and practitioner experiences of poorly performing horses found to have gastric ulceration. However, given the high prevalence of gastric ulcers in performance horses it should come as no surprise that ulcers are frequently found in poorly performing subjects. Subsequent improvement in performance following treatment is perhaps more convincing of a 'cause and effect' relationship (Mitchell, 2001; Johnson *et al.*, 2001; Franklin *et al.*, 2008), especially in the light of evidence suggesting no performance enhancing effect of omeprazole therapy (McKeever *et al.*, 2006), but could still be confounded by many other factors such as time, rest, dietary intake, bodyweight changes, other management changes or placebo effect. Large, controlled studies associating gastric ulcers with objective parameters of performance and subsequent response to specific therapy have not yet been published.

The majority of performance horses found to have gastric ulcers do not show readily detectable signs of pain (colic) although that is not to say that subclinical discomfort is not experienced by affected animals. Low grade abdominal pain is hard to detect and define in horses yet it seems likely that, if present, performance would indeed be compromised. Adverse GI related symptoms such as nausea, fullness/bloating and abdominal cramps have been shown to be quantitatively associated with impaired performance and power in human cyclists (Thorburn *et al.*, 2006).

Postoperative nutrition and condition

The energy needs of horses after colic or abdominal surgery are not known. Because of the wide variation in the severity of colic, clinicians have assumed that there is no need for an increase in nutritional requirement after simple colic. In most cases horses are only off feed for a short period of time (12-48 hours) if at all and there is no apparent clinical effect in these horses. Hypertriglyceridaemia has been documented in clinically ill horses with GI disease suggesting malnutrition occurs during periods without enteral nutrition and altered metabolism due to disease (Durham *et al.*, 2004). Sixteen Mcal (67 MJ; 32 kcal/kg), the energy requirement for maintenance for an adult horse on pasture, may not be needed for many horses that are stall confined and considered to have basal metabolism. During the immediate postoperative period as much as 15-20% less energy should be expended for digestion (Geor, 2007). The basal requirement for the stall confined horse postoperatively is likely sufficient unless they are challenged by a systemic inflammatory response syndrome due to peritonitis or endotoxemia. If the basal requirement is 70% of maintenance, the requirement for the stall rested horse would be approximately 21 kcal/kg per day (Geor 2007). Estimates for the increased energy requirement for horses due to abdominal surgery or shock are based on human information, which suggests an increase of 30% to 100% above maintenance, but this has not been substantiated in the horse. The protein requirement for maintenance is estimated at 1.25 g/kg per day providing 0.9 g/kg per day of available protein. Basal requirements for protein may also be decreased to 0.6-0.8 g/kg per day. Adequate energy from carbohydrates or fat is needed to prevent utilization of protein for energy during nutritional therapy.

Most hay or grass fed to horses is not evaluated for nutrient content, so the daily energy and protein intake frequently is not known for horses during medical care. The use of pellet formed feeds such as Equine Senior® allows calculation of the energy and protein intake. Other total horse feed supplied as pellets are usually made partially from grains thereby increasing soluble carbohydrate concentrations. This may be appropriate for some horses after surgery, but this is dependent on concern for altering the flora with excess starch in the caecum and colon and also perhaps stress induced insulin resistance and glucose intolerance. In some instances this readily available source of carbohydrates may be an advantage. Nevertheless, feedstuffs such as bran are not recommended due to the high amount of carbohydrate often present after milling (White, 2006).

Though not currently recognized as the standard of care, horses that are not ingesting at least 50% of their maintenance requirement (15-18 kcal/kg per day) for 48-72 hours should have nutritional support. Supplementation for severe GI disease has been used to increase survival and potentially limit the time required to return equine athletes to competition. Oral liquid diets made for humans have been used in horses for enteral nutrition but contain little fibre and increase the risk of colitis and laminitis. Other diets consisting of alfalfa pellets, dextrose, vegetable oils and amino acids maintained horses' weight but also increased the risk of diarrhoea and laminitis. Development of an enteral energy/protein source, which is readily absorbed with minimal risk of disturbing motility or gut flora is needed for horses requiring enteral nutrition during the initial post operative period. Supplementation of glutamine has been suggested to help maintain or restore the intestinal epithelium, reduce the inflammatory response of the epithelium, and prevent bacterial translocation (Zhang *et al.*, 1995; Blikslager *et al.*, 1999; Liboni *et al.*, 2005).

After a period of critical care for GI disease which involves prolonged ileus, shock or infection, horses commonly lose weight and muscle mass. The few studies that have measured the effect of severe disease on nutrition have not provided an objective measure of body condition. In the authors' experience is it not unusual for horses to lose 25-50 kg after prolonged treatment for colic or colitis. Though both inflammation and healing of the intestine is generally rapid, return to exercise and performance is determined by the horse's condition or in the case of abdominal surgery by healing of the abdominal wall.

Feeding horses intravenously though shown to be possible has not been proven to be necessary to improve horse survival after abdominal surgery. In human patients there is no evidence that parenteral nutrition alters mortality of surgical or critical care patients, but there is evidence that complications are decreased particularly in patients that are malnourished. A comparison of horses evaluated after abdominal surgery with or without supportive parenteral nutrition, did not show a difference in outcome. Nevertheless there was evidence of significantly decreased triglycerides, total bilirubin, albumin, and urea with significantly higher serum glucose and insulin in horses treated with parenteral nutrition after small intestinal resection and anastomosis (Durham *et al.*, 2004). The treatment did not change time until enteral feeding, time or cost of hospitalization. Parenteral nutrition should be considered immediately, if ileus, shock, or peritonitis is predicted to prevent oral ingestion of feed for more than a few days. Subjectively, it appears to the author that parenteral nutrition has been responsible for reducing convalescence time and cost for horses in shock and unable to tolerate enteral nutrition immediately after surgery. Parenteral supplementation may decrease weight loss and lessen the overall time required to rehabilitate horses for competition. Clearly more research in the area of nutrition for horses in need of critical care is required.

Intestinal surgery and performance

Equine intestine heals rapidly after enterotomy, or resection and anastomosis. The limiting factor for performance is normally the abdominal incision, which requires 2-4 months to heal and strengthen depending on the horse's postoperative and nutritional status. Though intestinal inflammation can be present for several weeks after surgery, the healing is normally rapid (Freeman *et al.*, 1988). Resection of greater than 60 percent of the small intestine has created nutritional compromise from lack of absorptive capacity with resultant poor body condition. Resection of the large colon can result in altered nutritional status including decreased phosphorus digestion. However, anecdotal observations suggest that after a period of adaptation horses can be successful in numerous types of performance after large colon resection. There appears to be a similar response to bypass of the ileum or the caecum. In both instances most reports success is defined as survival and the ability to compete not included (Ford *et al.*, 1990; Gerard *et al.*, 1996; Lores and Ortenburger, 2008). In the author's (NAW) experience the response to these techniques does not decrease a horse's ability to perform unless the original condition creates chronic inflammation or obstruction.

Colopexy which has been used to prevent large colon displacement or volvulus in horses is considered to be a high risk by surgically adhering the right, left or sternal flexure to the abdominal wall. The technique can be completed electively by laparoscopy, but there is hesitancy to complete the surgery in horses used for athletic competition due to the risk of colon rupture at the site of adhesion. Though anecdotal reports suggest horses can compete in events, a risk for fatal rupture does exist. In horses considered to have a high risk of recurrent colon displacement and that will be used for competition, colon resection is considered the best option.

Incisional hernia and performance

Abdominal or GI related problems that can limit performance after abdominal surgery include chronic obstruction, decreased absorptive capacity or incisional hernia. Except in cases of intestinal strangulation in the epiploic foramen, risk of death due to the original problem is not increased beyond 2 months after surgery. Though secondary colic risk is increased after abdominal surgery (Cohen *et al.*, 1995b) there is no report that indicates a decreased performance for a particular equine competition after surgery for colic.

The incidence of incisional hernia after ventral midline celiotomy in horses has been reported to range from 5.7-18% (Kobluk *et al.*, 1989). Studies have also reported that the risk of incisional hernia increases with relaparotomy, increased pain on recovery, leucopaenia, wound infection and high PCV (Gibson *et al.*, 1989; French *et al.*, 2002). As many as 20% of horses that develop incisional hernias have multiple smaller hernias along the incision (Gibson *et al.*, 1989) and may not require surgical intervention and can often be managed conservatively even for competition.

Ultrasound may be useful in the evaluation of the hernia. Adhesion of intestine to the hernial sac can complicate surgery or may be a risk for intestinal rupture during certain types of competition though this has not been documented. If surgical repair is required adequate time for maturation of the hernia ring and separated abdominal wall is required for adequate tissue strength for sutures. A minimum of three months is considered necessary after the initial surgery or when any infection has been controlled.

If the abdominal wall can be apposed primary closure should be completed. If the abdominal wall cannot be apposed, the hernia should be repaired using a synthetic mesh and fascial overlay using a horizontal or vertical mattress suture (Stick, 2006). Though no reports specify results of hernia repair by either method, anecdotal evidence suggests that there is no limitation after satisfactory healing.

Conclusions

The equine GI tract appears best adapted to a slow and constant intake of a high-fibre, low cereal diet. Optimal behavioural conditions for digestion, fermentation and assimilation of this diet are, most probably, a calm and restful state. Success in competition often demands restricted access to grazing and forage, feeding large quantities of cereal or fat, frequent bouts of intense or prolonged exercise, vehicular transport for long distances and relatively long periods of total feed deprivation. The GI tract responds to this adverse dietary management and exercise-associated stress with alterations in GI perfusion, motility, secretion, permeability and absorption. Frequent reports of exercise-associated GI symptoms in human athletes and also GI disease in several species suggests that the GI tract is not well adapted to an athletic career although evidence suggests that training may mitigate against the adverse effects of exertion. Colic or abdominal disease including the response to surgery, once resolved, does not limit a horse's potential for multiple forms of performance.

References

Abel, F.L., 1989. Myocardial function in sepsis and endotoxin shock. Am. J. Physiol. 257: R1265-R1281.

Aldoori, W.H., E.L. Giovannucci, E.B. Rimm, A. Ascherio, M.J. Stampfer, G.A. Colditz, A.L. Wing, D.V. Trichopoulos and W.C. Willett, 1995. Prospective study of physical activity and the risk of symptomatic diverticular disease in men.Gut. 36: 276-282.

Andrews, F.M. and J.A. Nadeau, 1999. Clinical syndromes of gastric ulceration in foals and mature horses. Equine Vet J Suppl. 29: 30-33.

Andrews, F.M., B.R. Buchanan, S.H. Smith, S.B. Elliott and A.M. Saxton, 2006. *In vitro* effects of hydrochloric acid and various concentrations of acetic, propionic, butyric, or valeric acids on bioelectric properties of equine gastric *squamous mucosa*. Am J Vet Res. 67: 1873-82.

Archer, D.C. and C.J. Proudman, 2006. Epidemiological clues to preventing colic. Vet J. 172: 29-39.

Argenzio, R.A., 1999. Comparative pathophysiology of nonglandular ulcer disease: a review of experimental studies. Equine Vet J Suppl. 29: 19-23.

Auer, D.E., K.V. Skelton, S. Tay and F.C. Baldock, 1993. Detection of bicarbonate administration (milkshake) in standardbred horses. Aust Vet J. 70: 336-340.

Bailey, S.R., A. Rycroft and J. Elliott, 2002. Production of amines in equine cecal contents in an in vitro model of carbohydrate overload. Journal of animal science 80: 2656-2662.

Bailey, S.R., C.M. Marr and J. Elliott, 2003. Identification and quantification of amines in the equine caecum. Research in veterinary science 74: 113-118.

Baker, B, S.L. Gaffin, M. Wells, B.C. Wessels and J.G. Brock-Utne, 1988. Endotoxaemia in racehorses following exertion. J S Afr Vet Assoc. 59: 63-66.

Barton, M.H., L. Williamson, S. Jacks and N. Norton, 2003. Effects on plasma endotoxin and eicosanoid concentrations and serum cytokine activities in horses competing in a 48-, 83-, or 159-km endurance ride under similar terrain and weather conditions. Am J Vet Res. 64: 754-761.

Begg, L.M. and C.B. O'Sullivan, 2003. The prevalence and distribution of gastric ulceration in 345 racehorses. Aust Vet J. 81: 199-201.

Bell, R.J.W., J.K. Kingston, T.D. Mogg and N.R. Perkins, 2007a. The prevalence of gastric ulceration in racehorses in New Zealand. N Z Vet J. 55: 13-18.

Bell, R.J.W., T.D. Mogg and J.K. Kingston, 2007b. Equine gastric ulcer syndrome in adult horses: a review. N Z Vet J. 55: 1-12.

Berschneider, H.M., A.T. Blikslager and M.C. Roberts, 1999. Role of duodenal reflux in nonglandular gastric ulcer disease of the mature horse. Equine Vet J Suppl. 29: 24-29.

Bertone, J.J., 2000. Prevalence of gastric ulcers in elite, heavy use western performance horses. Proc. Am. Assoc. Equine Pract. 46: 256-259.

Bi, L. and G. Triadafilopoulos, 2003. Exercise and GI function and disease: an evidence-based review of risks and benefits. Clin Gastroenterol Hepatol. 1: 345-55.

Bishop, R., 2005. Preparing and feeding the competition horse. Proc BEVA Waltham Nutr Symp 1: 141-146.

Blikslager, A.T., J.M. Rhoads, D.G. Bristol, M.C. Roberts and R.A. Argenzio, 1999. Glutamine and transforming growth factor-alpha stimulate extracellular regulated kinases and enhance recovery of villous surface area in porcine ischemic-injured intestine. Surgery. 125: 186-194.

Bosenberg, A.T., J.G. Brock-Utne, S.L. Gaffin, M.T. Wells and G.T. Blake, 1988. Strenuous exercise causes systemic endotoxemia. J Appl Physiol. 65: 106-108.

Brouns, F. and E. Beckers, 1993. Is the gut an athletic organ? Digestion, absorption and exercise. Sports Med.15: 242-257.

Bueno, A.C., T.L. Seahorn and R.M. Moore, 2000. Diagnosis and treatment of right, dorsal colitis in horses. Compend Contin Educ Pract Vet. 22: 173-175.

Butudom, P., S.M. Axiak, B.D. Nielsen, S.W. Eberhart and H.C. Schott Jr., 2003. Effect of varying initial drink volume on rehydration of horses. Physiology & behavior 79, 135-142.

Campbell-Thompson, M.L. and A.M. Merritt, 1990. Basal and pentagastrin-stimulated gastric secretion in young horses. Am J Physiol. 259: R1259-R1266.

Camus, G., J. Poortmans, M. Nys, G. Deby-Dupont, J. Duchateau, C. Deby and M. Lamy, 1997. Mild endotoxaemia and the inflammatory response induced by a marathon race. Clin Sci (Lond). 92: 415-422.

Cannon, J.G. and M.J. Kluger, 1983. Endogenous pyrogen activity in human plasma after exercise. Science 220: 617-619.

Cargile, J.L., J.A. Burrow, I. Kim, N.D. Cohen and A.M. Merritt, 2004. Effect of dietary corn oil supplementation on equine gastric fluid acid, sodium, and prostaglandin E2 content before and during pentagastrin infusion. J Vet Intern Med. 18: 545-549.

Carlson, G.P. and R.A. Mansmann, 1974. Serum electrolyte and plasma protein alterations in horses used in endurance rides. J Am Vet Med Assoc 165: 262-264.

Carrió, I., M. Estorch, R. Serra-Grima, M. Ginjaume, R. Notivol, R. Calabuig and F. Vilardell, 1989. Gastric emptying in marathon runners. Gut. 30: 152-155.

Choi, S.C., S.J. Choi, J.A. Kim, T.H. Kim, Y.H. Nah, E. Yazaki and D.F. Evans, 2001. The role of GI endoscopy in long-distance runners with GI symptoms. Eur J Gastroenterol Hepatol. 13: 1089-1094.

Choi, S.J., Y.S. Kim, J.R. Chae, H.K. Cho, T.H. Kim, Y.W. Sohn, Y.L. Oh, G.S. Seo, Y.H. Nah and S.C. Choi, 2006. Effects of ranitidine for exercise induced gastric mucosal changes and bleeding. World J Gastroenterol. 12: 2579-2583

Clarke, L.L., M.C. Roberts and R.A. Argenzio, 1990. Feeding and digestive problems in horses. Vet Clin North Am Equine Pract. 6: 319-337.

Clausen, J.P., 1997. Effect of physical training on cardiovascular adjustments to exercise in man. Physiol Rev 57: 779-815.

Cohen, N.D., 2002. Right dorsal colitis. Equine Vet Educ. 14: 212-219

Cohen, N.D. and J.G. Peloso, 1996. Risk factors for history of previous colic and for chronic, intermittent colic in a population of horses. J Am Vet Med Assoc. 208: 697-703.

Cohen, N.D., G.K. Carter, R.H. Mealey and T.S. Taylor, 1995a. Medical management of right dorsal colitis in 5 horses: a retrospective study (1987-1993). J Vet Intern Med. 9: 272-276.

Cohen, N.D., P.L. Matejka, C.M. Honnas and R.N. Hooper, 1995b. Case-control study of the association between various management factors and development of colic in horses. Texas Equine Colic Study Group. J Am Vet Med Assoc. 206: 667-673.

Cohen, N.D., P.G. Gibbs and A.M. Woods, 1999. Dietary and other management factors associated with colic in horses. J Am Vet Med Assoc. 215: 53-60.

Cohen, N.D., E. Toby, A.J. Roussel, E.L. Murphey and N. Wang, 2006. Are feeding practices associated with duodenitis-proximal jejunitis? Equine Vet J. 38: 526-531.

Cox, R., C.J. Proudman, A.F. Trawford, F. Burden and G.L. Pinchbeck, 2007. Epidemiology of impaction colic in donkeys in the UK. BMC Vet Res. 3: 1.

Cuddeford, D., 2000. The significance of pH in the hind gut. Proc Dodson & Horrell Int Conf. Feeding horses 3: 3-9.

Dabareiner, R.M. and N.A. White, 1995. Large colon impaction in horses: 147 cases (1985-1991). J Am Vet Med Assoc. 206: 679-685.

Dart, A.J., J.R. Snyder, S.J. Spier and K.E. Sullivan, 1992. Ionized calcium concentration in horses with surgically managed gastrointestinal disease: 147 cases (1988-1990). J Am Vet Med Assoc 201, 1244-1248.

Davis, M.S., M.D. Willard, K.K. Williamson, J.M. Steiner and D.A. Williams, 2005. Sustained strenuous exercise increases intestinal permeability in racing Alaskan sled dogs. J Vet Intern Med. 19: 34-39.

Davis, M., M. Willard, K. Williamson, C. Royer, M. Payton, J.M. Steiner, K. Hinchcliff, E. McKenzie and S. Nelson, 2006. Temporal relationship between gastrointestinal protein loss, gastric ulceration or erosion, and strenuous exercise in racing Alaskan sled dogs. J Vet Intern Med. 20: 835-839.

De Fombelle, A., V. Julliand, C. Drogoul and E. Jacotot, 2001. Feeding and microbial disorders in horses: 1-Effects of an abrupt incorporation of two levels of barley in a hay diet on microbial profile and activities. J Eq Vet Sci. 26: 439-445.

De Lira, C.A., R.L. Vancini, S.S. Ihara, A.C. da Silva, J. Aboulafia and V.L. Nouailhetas, 2008. Aerobic exercise affects C57BL/6 murine intestinal contractile function. Eur J Appl Physiol. 103: 215-23.

Demers, L.M., T.S. Harrison, D.R. Halbert and R.J. Santen, 1981. Effect of prolonged exercise on plasma prostaglandin levels. Prostaglandins Med. 6: 413-418.

De Schryver, A.M., Y.C. Keulemans, H.P. Peters, L.M. Akkermans, A.J. Smout, W.R. De Vries and G.P. van Berge-Henegouwen, 2005. Effects of regular physical activity on defecation pattern in middle-aged patients complaining of chronic constipation. Scand J Gastroenterol. 40: 422-429.

Dionne, R.M., A. Vrins, M.Y. Doucet and J. Paré, 2003. Gastric ulcers in standardbred racehorses: prevalence, lesion description, and risk factors. J Vet Intern Med. 17: 218-222.

Drogoul, C., A. de Fombelle and V. Julliand, 2001. Feeding and microbial disorders in horses: 2: Effect of three hay:grain ratios on digesta passage rate and digestibility in ponies. J Eq Vet Sci. 26: 487-491.

Durham, A.E., 2007. The role of nutrition in colic. In: A. Lindner (Ed) Applied equine nutrition and training, Proceedings of the Equine Nutrition Conference (ENUCO), Wageningen Academic Publishers, Wageningen, the Netherlands pp. 79-93.

Durham, A.E., T.J. Phillips, J.P. Walmsley and JR. Newton, 2004. Nutritional and clinicopathological effects of post operative parenteral nutrition following small intestinal resection and anastomosis in the mature horse. Equine Vet J 36: 390-396.

Ellis, J.M., T. Hollands and D.E. Allen, 2002. Effect of forage intake on bodyweight and performance. Equine Vet J Suppl. 34: 66-70.

Equine Gastric Ulcer Council, 1999. Recommendations for the diagnosis and treatment of equine gastric ulcer syndrome (EGUS). Equine Vet Educ. 11: 262-272.

Ethell, M.T., D.R. Hodgson and B.A. Hills, 2000. Evidence for surfactant contributing to the gastric mucosal barrier of the horse. Equine Vet J. 32: 470-474.

Fink, M.P., K.L. Kaups, H.L. Wang and H.R. Rothschild, 1991. Maintenance of superior mesenteric arterial perfusion prevents increased intestinal mucosal permeability in endotoxic pigs. Surgery. 110: 154-160.

Foreman, J.H., 1998. The exhausted horse syndrome. The Veterinary clinics of North America 14, 205-219.

Frank, N, F.M. Andrews, S.B. Elliott and J. Lew, 2005. Effects of dietary oils on the development of gastric ulcers in mares. Am J Vet Res. 66: 2006-2011.

Franklin, S.H., T.J. Brazil and K.J. Allen, 2008. Poor performance associated with equine gastric ulceration syndrome in four Thoroughbred racehorses. Equine Vet Educ. 20: 119-124.

Freeman, D.E., R.E. Cimprich, D.W. Richardson, D.G. Gentile, J.A. Orsini, E.P. Tulleners and J.P. Fetrow, 1988. Early mucosal healing and chronic changes in pony jejunum after various types of strangulation obstruction. Am J Vet Res 49: 810-818.

French, N.P, J. Smith, G.B. Edwards and C.J. Proudman, 2002. Equine surgical colic: risk factors for postoperative complications. Equine Vet J 34: 444-449.

Ford, T.S., D.E. Freeman, M.W. Ross, D.W. Richardson, B.B. Martin and J.B. Madison, 1990. Ileocecal intussusception in horses: 26 cases (1981-1988). J Am Vet Med Assoc. 196, 121-126.

Furr, M.O., M.J. Murray and D.C. Ferguson, 1992. The effects of stress on gastric ulceration, T3, T4, reverse T3 and cortisol in neonatal foals. Equine Vet J. 24: 37-40.

Furr, M., L. Taylor and K. Kronfeld, 1994. The effects of exercise training on serum gastrin responses in the horse. Cornell Vet. 84: 41-45.

Garcia-Lopez, J.M., P.J. Provost, J.E. Rush, S.C. Zicker, H. Burmaster and L.M. Freeman, 2001. Prevalence and prognostic importance of hypomagnesemia and hypocalcemia in horses that have colic surgery. Am J Vet Res 62: 7-12.

Geor, R.J., 2000. Gastric surface active phospholipid – a role in protection of the squamous epithelial mucosa? Equine Vet J. 32: 458-459.

Geor, R.J., 2007. How to feed horses recovering from colic. Proceedings Ann Conv AAEP 52: 196-201.

Geor, R.J. and P.A. Harris, 2005. Nutritional management of endurance horses. Proc BEVA Waltham Nutr Symp 1: 71-77.

Geor, R.J. and P.A. Harris, 2007. How to minimize gastrointestinal disease associated with carbohydrate nutrition in horses. Proceedings Ann Conv AAEP 52, 178-185.

Geor, R.J., D.J. Weiss and C.M. Smith, 1994. Hemorheologic alterations induced by incremental treadmill exercise in thoroughbreds. Am J Vet Res. 55: 854-861.

Gerard, M.P., K.F. Bowman, A.T. Blikslager, L.P. Tate Jr and D.G. Bristol, 1996. Jejunocolostomy or ileocolostomy for treatment of cecal impaction in horses: nine cases (1985-1995). J Am Vet Med Assoc 209: 1287-1290.

Gibson, K.T., C.R. Curtis, A.S. Turner, C.W. McIlwraith, W.A. Aanes and T.S. Stashak, 1989. Incisional hernias in the horse. Incidence and predisposing factors. Vet Surg 18: 360-366.

Gil, S.M., E. Yazaki and D.F. Evans, 1998. Aetiology of running-related GI dysfunction. How far is the finishing line? Sports Med. 26: 365-378.

Gisolfi, C.V., 2000. Is the GI System Built For Exercise? News Physiol Sci. 15: 114-119.

Goodson, J., W.J. Tyznik, J.H. Cline and B.A. Dehority, 1988. Effects of an abrupt diet change from hay to concentrate on microbial numbers and physical environment in the cecum of the pony. Appl. Environ Microbiol. 54: 1946-1950.

Hall, G.M., T.E. Adrian, S.R. Bloom and J.N. Lucke, 1982. Changes in circulating gut hormones in the horse during long distance exercise. Equine Vet J. 14: 209-212.

Hammond, C.J., D.K. Mason and K.L. Watkins, 1986. Gastric ulceration in mature thoroughbred horses. Equine Vet J. 18: 284-287.

Hartmann, A.M. and R.L. Frankeny, 2003. A preliminary investigation into the association between competition and gastric ulcer formation in non-racing performance horses J Equine Vet Sci 23: 560-561.

Hess, T.M., D.S. Kronfeld, C.W. Williams, J.N. Waldron, P.M. Graham-Thiers, K. Greiwe-Crandell, M.A. Lopes and P.A. Harris, 2005. Effects of oral potassium supplementation on acid-base status and plasma ion concentrations of horses during endurance exercise. Am J Vet Res 66: 466-473.

Hillyer, M.H., F.G. Taylor and N.P. French, 2001. A cross-sectional study of colic in horses on thoroughbred training premises in the British Isles in 1997. Equine Vet J. 33: 380-385.

Hillyer, M.H., F.G. Taylor, C.J. Proudman, G.B. Edwards, J.E. Smith and N.P. French, 2002. Case control study to identify risk factors for simple colonic obstruction and distension colic in horses. Equine Vet J. 34: 455-463.

Hintz, H.F., 2000. Equine nutrition update. Proc Am Assoc Equine Pract. 46: 62-79.

Holbrook, T.C., R.D. Simmons, M.E. Payton and C.G. MacAllister, 2005. Effect of repeated oral administration of hypertonic electrolyte solution on equine gastric mucosa. Equine Vet J. 37: 501-504.

Houpt, K.A., 1990. Ingestive behaviour. Vet Clin North Am Equine Pract. 6: 319-337.

Hudson, J.M., N.D. Cohen, P.G. Gibbs and J.A. Thompson, 2001. Feeding practices associated with colic in horses. J Am Vet Med Assoc. 219: 1419-1425.

Hussein, H.S., L.A. Vogedes, G.C. Fernandez and R.L. Frankeny, 2004. Effects of cereal grain supplementation on apparent digestibility of nutrients and concentrations of fermentation end-products in the feces and serum of horses consuming alfalfa cubes. J Anim Sci. 82: 1986-1996.

Jansen, W.L., S.N.J. Geleen, J. van der Kuilen and A.C. Beynen, 2002. Dietary soyabean oil depresses the apparent digestibility of fibre in trotters when substituted for an iso-energetic amount of corn starch or glucose. Equine Vet J 34: 302-305.

Johnson, J.H., N. Vatistas, L. Castro, T. Fischer, F.S. Pipers and D. Maye, 2001. Fiedl survey of the prevalence of gastric ulcers in Thoroughbred racehorses and on response to treatment of affected horses with omperazole. Equine Vet Educ 13: 221-224.

Jonsson, H. and A. Egenvall, 2006. Prevalence of gastric ulceration in Swedish Standardbreds in race training. Equine Vet J. 38: 209-213.

Jozkow, P. D. Wasko-Czopnik, M. Medras and L. Paradowski, 2006. Gastroesophageal reflux disease and physical activity. Sports Med.36: 385-391.

Julliand, V., A. de Fombelle, C. Drogoul and E. Jacotot, 2001. Feeding and microbial disorders in horses: Part 3. Effects of three hay:grain ratios on microbial profile and activities. J Eq Vet Sci. 26: 543-546.

Kallings, P., 1993. Nonsteroidal anti-inflammatory drugs. Vet Clin North Am Equine Pract. 9: 523-541.

Kaneene, J.B., R. Miller, W.A. Ross, K. Gallagher, J. Marteniuk and J. Rook, 1997. Risk factors for colic in the Michigan (USA) equine population. Prev Vet Med. 30: 23-36.

Karcher, L.F., S.G. Dill, W.I. Anderson and J.M. King, 1990. Right dorsal colitis. J Vet Intern Med. 4: 247-253.

Klein, I., S. Reif, H. Farbstein, A. Halak and T. Gilat, 1998. Preillness non dietary factors and habits in inflammatory bowel disease. Ital J Gastroenterol Hepatol. 30: 247-251.

Kobluk, C.N., N.G. Ducharme, J.H. Lumsden, P.J. Pascoe, M.A Livesey, M. Hurtig, F.D. Horney and M. Arighi, 1989. Factors affecting incisional complication rates associated with colic surgery in horses: 78 cases (1983-1985). Journal of the American Veterinary Medical Association 195: 639-642.

Kronfeld, D.S., P.L. Ferrante and D. Grandjean, 1994. Optimal nutrition for athletic performance, with emphasis on fat adaptation in dogs and horses. J Nutr 124(12 Suppl): 2745S-2753S.

Kronfeld, D.S., 1996. Dietary fat affects heat production and other variables of equine performance, under hot and humid conditions. Equine veterinary journal, 24-34.

Lambert, G.P., M. Boylan, J.P. Laventure, A. Bull and S. Lanspa, 2007. Effect of aspirin and ibuprofen on GI permeability during exercise. Int J Sports Med. 28: 722-726.

Lang, J.A., C.V. Gisolfi and G.P. Lambert, 2006. Effect of exercise intensity on active and passive glucose absorption. Int. J Sport Nutr Exerc Metab. 16: 485-493.

Leiper, J.B., C.W. Nicholas, A. Ali, C. Williams and R.J. Maughan, 2005. The effect of intermittent high-intensity running on gastric emptying of fluids in man. Med. Sci Sports Exerc. 37: 240-247.

Le Jeune, S.S., J.E. Nieto, J.E. Dechant and JR. Snyder, 2006. Prevalence of gastric ulcers in Thoroughbred broodmares in pasture. Proc Am Assoc Equine Pract. 52: 264.

Liboni, K.C., N. Li, P.O. Scumpia and J. Neu, 2005. Glutamine modulates LPS-induced IL-8 production through IkappaB/NF-kappaB in human fetal and adult intestinal epithelium. J Nutr. 135: 245-251.

Lichtenberger, L.M., Y. Zhou, E.J. Dial, R.M. Raphael, 2006. NSAID injury to the gastrointestinal tract: evidence that NSAIDs interact with phospholipids to weaken the hydrophobic surface barrier and induce the formation of unstable pores in membranes. J Pharm Pharmacol. 58: 1421-1428.

Lopes, M.A., N.A. White, M.V. Crisman and D.L. Ward, 2004. Effects of feeding large amounts of grain on colonic contents and feces in horses. Am J Vet Res 65(5): 687-94.

Lorenzo-Figueras, M. and A.M. Merritt, 2002. Effects of exercise on gastric volume and pH in the proximal portion of the stomach of horses. Am J Vet Res. 65: 687-694.

Lores, M. and A.I. Ortenburger, 2008. Use of cecal bypass via side-to-side ileocolic anastomosis without ileal transection for treatment of cecocolic intussusception in three horses. J Am Vet Med Assoc 232: 574-577.

Love, S., M.H. Hillyer, D.M. Murphy and S.W.J. Reid, 1994. Historical and clinical data from 39 cases of colonic (pelvic flexure) impaction. Proc Equine Colic Res Symp 5:36-37.

Lucas, W. and P.C. Schroy, 1998. Reversible ischemic colitis in a high endurance athlete. Am J Gastroenterol 93: 2231-2334.

Lybbert, T., P. Gibbs, N. Cohen, B. Scott and D. Sigler, 2007. Feeding alfalfa hay to exercising horses reduces the severity of gastric squamous mucosal ulceration. Proc Am Assoc Equine Pract. 53: 525-526.

Manohar, M., 1986. Blood flow to the respiratory and limb muscles and to abdominal organs during maximal exertion in ponies. J Physiol. 377: 25-35.

Manohar, M., T.E. Goetz, B. Saupe, E. Hutchens and E. Coney, 1995. Thyroid, renal, and splanchnic circulation in horses at rest and during short-term exercise. Am J Vet Res. 56: 1356-1361.

Mansmann, R.A., G.P. Carlson, N.A. White and D.W. Milne, 1974. Synchronous diaphragmatic flutter in horses. J Am Vet Med Assoc 165(3): 265-70

Martin, B.B., V.B. Reef, E.J. Parente and A.D. Sage, 2000. Causes of poor performance of horses during training, racing, or showing: 348 cases (1992-1996). J Am Vet Med Assoc. 216: 554-558.

Matsumoto, M., R. Inoue, T. Tsukahara, K. Ushida, H. Chiji, N. Matsubara and H. Hara, 2008. Voluntary running exercise alters microbiota composition and increases n-butyrate concentration in the rat cecum. Biosci Biotechnol Biochem. 72: 572-576.

McClure, S.R., L.T. Glickman and N.W. Glickman, 1999. Prevalence of gastric ulcers in show horses. J. Am. Vet. Med. Assoc. 215: 1130-1133.

McClure, S.R., D.S. Carithers, S.J. Gross and M.J. Murray, 2005. Gastric ulcer development in horses in a simulated show or training environment. J Am Vet Med Assoc. 227: 775-777.

McConnico, R.S., R.M. Moore and J.D. Hubert, 2006. Right dorsal colonic pathophyisology in horses administered Phenylbutazone, 2006 Equine Research Report, Louisiana State University, pp 35-36.

McCutcheon, L.J. and R.J. Geor, 1998. Sweating. Fluid and ion losses and replacement. Vet Clinics of N Am: Equine 14: 75-95.

McCutcheon, L.J., R.J. Geor, G.L. Ecker and M.I. Lindinger, 1999. Equine sweating responses to submaximal exercise during 21 days of heat acclimation. J Appl Physiol 87: 1843-1851.

McKeever, J.M., K.H. McKeever, J.M. Albeirci, M.E. Gordon and H.C. Manso Filho, 2006. Effect of omeprazole on markers of performance in gastric ulcer-free standardbred horses. Equine Vet J Suppl. 36: 668-671.

Merritt, A.M., 1999. Normal equine gastroduodenal secretion and motility. Equine Vet J. Suppl. 29: 7-13.

Merritt, A.M., 2003. The equine stomach: a personal perspective (1963-2003). Proc Am Assoc Equine Pract. 49: 75-102.

Metayer, N, M. Lhote, A. Bahr, N.D. Cohen, I. Kim, A.J. Roussel and V. Julliand, 2004. Meal size and starch content affect gastric emptying in horses. Equine Vet J. 36: 436-440.

Meyer, H., M. Coenen and C. Gurer, 1985. Investigations on saliva production and chewing effects in horses fed various feeds Proc. Equine Nutr. Physiol. Soc. 9: 38-41.

Mitchell, R.D., 2001. Prevalence of gastric ulcers in hunter/jumper and dressage horses evaluated for poor performance. Proc Assoc Equine Sports Med 21. http://gastrogard.us.merial.com/pix/pdf/MLEQ1022_PrevalanceGU_TB1.pdf Accessed 9th March 2008.

Monreal, L., D. Sabaté, D. Segura, I. Mayós and J. Homedes, 2004. Lower gastric ulcerogenic effect of suxibuzone compared to phenylbutazone when administered orally to horses. Res Vet Sci. 76: 145-149.

Morris, E.A. and H.J. Seeherman, 1991. Clinical evaluation of poor performance in the racehorse: the results of 275 evaluations. Equine Vet J.23: 169-174.

Moses, F.M., 1990. The effect of exercise on the GI tract. Sports Med. 9: 159-72.

Murray, M.J., 1992a. Aetiopathogenesis and treatment of peptic ulcer in the horse: a comparative review. Equine Vet J suppl. 13: 63-74.

Murray, M.J., 1992b. Gastric ulceration in horses: 91 cases (1987-1990). J Am Vet Med Assoc. 201: 117-120.

Murray, M.J., 1997. Suppression of gastric acidity in horses. J Am Vet Med Assoc. 211: 37-40.

Murray, M.J., 1999. Pathophysiology of peptic disorders in foals and horses: a review. Equine Vet J Suppl. 29: 14-18.

Murray, M.J. and E.S. Eichorn, 1996. Effects of intermittent feed deprivation, intermittent feed deprivation with ranitidine administration, and stall confinement with ad libitum access to hay on gastric ulceration in horses. Am J Vet Res. 57: 1599-1603.

Murray, M.J. and C. Grodinsky, 1989. Regional gastric pH measurement in horses and foals. Equine Vet J Suppl.7: 73-76.

Murray, M.J., C. Grodinsky, C.W. Anderson, P.F. Radue and G.R. Schmidt, 1989. Gastric ulcers in horses: a comparison of endoscopic findings in horses with and without clinical signs. Equine Vet J Suppl. 7: 68-72.

Murray, M.J., G.F. Schusser, F.S. Pipers and S.J. Gross, 1996. Factors associated with gastric lesions in thoroughbred racehorses. Equine Vet J. 28: 368-74.

Murray, M.J., Y.S. Nout and D.L. Ward, 2001. Endoscopic findings of the gastric antrum and pylorus in horses: 162 cases (1996-2000). J Vet Intern Med.15: 401-406.

Nadeau, J.A., F.M. Andrews, A.G. Mathew, R.A. Argenzio, J.T. Blackford, M. Sohtell and A.M. Saxton, 2000. Evaluation of diet as a cause of gastric ulcers in horses. Am J Vet Res. 61: 784-790.

Nadeau, J.A., F.M. Andrews, C.S. Patton, R.A. Argenzio, A.G. Mathew and A.M. Saxton, 2003a. Effects of hydrochloric, acetic, butyric, and propionic acids on pathogenesis of ulcers in the nonglandular portion of the stomach of horses. Am J Vet Res. 64: 404-412.

Nadeau, J.A., F.M. Andrews, C.S. Patton, R.A. Argenzio, A.G. Mathew and A.M. Saxton, 2003b. Effects of hydrochloric, valeric, and other volatile fatty acids on pathogenesis of ulcers in the nonglandular portion of the stomach of horses. Am J Vet Res. 64: 413-417.

Nagata, S., F. Takeda, M. Kurosawa, K. Mima, A. Hiraga, M. Kai and K. Taya, 1999. Plasma adrenocorticotropin, cortisol and catecholamines response to various exercises. Equine Vet J Suppl. 30: 570-574.

National Research Council, 2007a. Water and water quality. In: Nutrient Requirements of Horses, 6th edition, pp 128-140. National Academies Press, Washington.

National Research Council, 2007b. Feeding behavior and general considerations for feeding management. In: Nutrient Requirements of Horses, 6th edition, pp 211-234. National Academies Press, Washington.

Naylor, J.R., W.M. Bayly, H.C. Schott, P.D. Gollnick and D.R. Hodgson, 1993. Equine plasma and blood volumes decrease with dehydration but subsequently increase with exercise. J Appl Physiol 75: 1002-1008.

Neufer, P.D., A.J. Young, M.N. Sawka, 1989. Gastric emptying during walking and running: effects of varied exercise intensity. Eur J Appl Physiol Occup Physiol.58: 440-445.

Nieto, J.E., J.R. Snyder, P. Beldomenico, M. Aleman, J.W. Kerr and S.J. Spier, 2004. Prevalence of gastric ulcers in endurance horses - a preliminary report. Vet. J. 167: 33-37.

Nyman, S., A. Jansson, K. Dahlborn and A. Lindholm, 1996. Strategies for voluntary rehydration in horses during endurance exercise. Equine Vet J Suppl. 22: 99-106.

O'Connor, A.M., C.F. Johnston, K.D. Buchanan, C. Boreham, T.R. Trinick and C.J. Riddoch, 1995. Circulating GI hormone changes in marathon running. Int J Sports Med. 16: 283-287.

Olsson, N. and A. Ruudvere, 1955. The nutrition of the horse. Nutr Abstr Rev Ser Hum Exp. 25: 1-18.

Orton, R.K., I.D. Hume and R.A. Leng, 1985a. Effects of level of dietary protein and exercise on growth rates of horses. Equine Vet J. 17: 381-385.

Orton, R.K., I.D. Hume and R.A. Leng, 1985b. Effects of exercise and level of dietary protein on digestive function in horses. Equine Vet J. 17: 386-390.

Pagan, J.D., P. Harris, T. Brewster-Barnes, S.E. Duren and S.G. Jackson, 1998. Exercise affects digestibility and rate of passage of all-forage and mixed diets in Thoroughbred horses. J Nutr 128: 2704S-2707S.

Pagan, J.D. and P.A. Harris, 1999. The effects of timing and amount of forage and grain on exercise response in thoroughbred horses. Equine Vet J Suppl 30: 451-7.

Pals, K.L., R.T. Chang, A.J. Ryan and C.V. Gisolfi, 1997. Effect of running intensity on intestinal permeability. J Appl Physiol. 82: 571-576.

Pearson, R.A. and J.B. Merritt, 1991. Intake, digestion and GI transit time in resting donkeys and ponies and exercised donkeys given ad libitum hay and straw diets. Equine Vet J. 23: 339-343.

Peters, H.P., W.C. Wiersma, L.M. Akkermans, E. Bol, R.J. Kraaijenhagen, W.L. Mosterd, W.R. de Vries and J.P. Wielders, 2000a. GI mucosal integrity after prolonged exercise with fluid supplementation. Med Sci Sports Exerc. 32: 134-142.

Peters, H.P., J.W. Wiersma, J. Koerselman, L.M. Akkermans, E. Bol, W.L. Mosterd and W.R. de Vries, 2000b. The effect of a sports drink on gastroesophageal reflux during a run-bike-run test. Int J Sports Med. 21: 65-70.

Peters, H.P., W.R. de Vries, G.P. Vanberge-Henegouwen and L.M. Akkermans, 2001. Potential benefits and hazards of physical activity and exercise on the GI tract. Gut 48: 435-439.

Potter, G.D., F.F. Arnold, D.D. Householder, D.H. Hansen and K.M. Brown, 1992. Digestion of starch in the small or large intestine of the equine. Europische Konferenz uber die Ernahrung des Pferdes. PferdeHeilkunde Sonderheft 1: 107-111.

Rabuffo, T.S., J.A. Orsini, E. Sullivan, J. Engiles, T. Norman and R. Boston, 2002. Associations between age or sex and prevalence of gastric ulceration in Standardbred racehorses in training. J. Am. Vet. Med. Assoc. 221: 1156-1159.

Reed, S.K., N.T. Messer, R.K. Tessman and K.G. Keegan, 2006. Effects of phenylbutazone alone or in combination with flunixin meglumine on blood protein concentrations in horses. Am J Vet Res. 67: 398-402.

Reeves, M.J., M.D. Salman and G. Smith, 1996. Risk factors for equine acute abdominal disease (colic): results from a multi-center case-control study. Prev. Vet. Med. 26: 285-301.

Rehrer, N.J. and G.A. Meijer, 1991. Biomechanical vibration of the abdominal region during running and bicycling. J Sports Med Phys Fitness 31: 231-234.

Rehrer, N.J., E.J. Beckers, F. Brouns, F. ten Hoor and W.H. Saris, 1990. Effects of dehydration on gastric emptying and GI distress while running. Med Sci Sports Exerc 22: 790- 795.

Rice, O., R. Geor, P. Harris, K. Hoekstra, S. Gardners and J. Pagan, 2001. Effects of restricted hay intake on bodyweight and metabolic responses to high-intesity exercise in Thoroughbred horses. Proc equine Nutr Physiol Symp 17: 273-279.

Richards, N., G. Hinch and J. Rowe, 2006. The effect of current grain feeding practices on hindgut starch fermentation and acidosis in the Australian racing Thoroughbred. Aust Vet J. 84: 402-407.

Rosa, E.F., E. Freymuller, S.S. Ihara, J. Aboulafia and V.L. Nouailhetas, 2008. Damaging effects of intense repetitive treadmill running on murine intestinal musculature. J Appl Physiol. 104: 1410-1417.

Rose, R.J. and D.R. Lloyd, 1992. Sodium bicarbonate: more than just a 'milkshake'? Equine Vet J. 24: 75-76.

Rose, R.J., K.S. Arnold, S. Church and R. Paris, 1980. Plasma and sweat electrolyte concentrations in the horse during long distance exercise. Equine Vet J 12: 19-22.

Sakurada, S. and J.R. Hales, 1998. A role for GI endotoxins in enhancement of heat tolerance by physical fitness. J Appl Physiol. 84: 207-214.

Sanchez, L.D., B. Corwell and D. Berkoff, 2006. Medical problems of marathon runners. Am J Emerg Med 24: 608-615L.

Sandin, A., K. Girma, B. Sjöholm, A. Lindholm and G. Nilsson, 1998. Effects of differently composed feeds and physical stress on plasma gastrin concentration in horses. Acta Vet Scand. 39: 265-272.

Simons, S.M. and R.G. Kennedy, 2004. Gastrointestinal problems in runners. Curr Sports Med Rep. 3: 112-116.

Simrén, M., 2002. Physical activity and the GI tract. Eur J Gastroenterol Hepatol. 14: 1053-1056.

Smetanka, R.D., G.P. Lambert, R. Murray, D. Eddy, M. Horn and C.V. Gisolfi, 1999. Intestinal permeability in runners in the 1996 Chicago Marathon. Int J Sport Nutr. 9: 426-433.

Smyth, G.B., D.W. Young and L.S. Hammond, 1989. Effects of diet and feeding on postprandial serum gastrin and insulin concentration in adult horses. Equine Vet J Suppl. 7: 56-59.

Sosa León, L.A., D.R. Hodgson and R.J. Rose, 1997. Gastric emptying of oral rehydration solutions at rest and after exercise in horses. Res Vet Sci. 63: 183-187.

Stämpfli, H. and O.E. Oliver, 2006. Chronic diarrhea and weight loss in three horses. Vet Clin North Am Equine Pract. 22: e27-35 (http://download.journals.elsevierhealth.com/pdfs/journals/0749-0739/PIIS0749073905000994.pdf Accessed 8-Mar-2008).

Stick, J.A., 2006. Abdominal Hernias. In: J.A. Auer and J.A. Stick (Eds.) Equine Surgery, 3rd edition. St Louis: Saunders Elsevier; p. 495.

Sullivan, S.N., 1987. Exercise-associated symptoms in traithletes. Phys Sports Med 15: 105-108.

Sullivan, S.N. and C. Wong, 1992. Runners' diarrhea. Different patterns and associated factors. J Clin Gastroenterol.14: 101-104.

Thorburn, M.S., B. Vistisen, R.M. Thorp, M.J. Rockell, A.E. Jeukendrup, X. Xu and D.S. Rowlands, 2006. Attenuated gastric distress but no benefit to performance with adaptation to octanoate-rich esterified oils in well-trained male cyclists. J Appl Physiol. 101: 1733-1743.

Thune, I. and A.S. Furberg, 2001. Physical activity and cancer risk: dose-response and cancer, all sites and site-specific. Med Sci Sports Exerc. 33: S530-S550.

Tinker, M.K., N.A. White, P. Lessard, C.D. Thatcher, K.D. Pelzer, B. Davis and D.K. Carmel, 1997. A prospective study of equine colic incidence and mortality. Equine Vet J. 29: 448-453.

Traub-Dargatz, J.L., C.A. Kopral, A.H. Seitzinger, L.P. Garber, K. Forde and N.A. White, 2001. Estimate of the national incidence of and operation-level risk factors for colic among horses in the United State, spring 1998 to spring 1999. J Am Vet Med Assoc. 219: 67-71.

Treiber, K.H., T.M. Hess, D.S. Kronfeld, R.C. Boston, R.J. Geor, M. Friere, A.M. Silva and P.A. Harris, 2006. Glucose dynamics during exercise: dietary energy sources affect minimal model parameters in trained Arabian geldings during endurance exercise. Equine Vet J Suppl: 631-636.

Vatistas, N.J., J.R. Snyder, G. Carlson, B. Johnson, R.M. Arthur, M. Thurmond and K.C.K. Lloyd, 1994. Epidemiological study of gastric ulceration in the Thoroughbred race horse: 202 horses 1992-1993. Proc Am Assoc Equine Pract 40: 125-126.

Vatistas, N.J., R.L. Sifferman, J. Holste, J.L. Cox, G. Pinalto and K.T. Schultz, 1999a. Induction and maintenance of gastric ulceration in horses in simulated race training. Equine Vet J Suppl 29: 40-44.

Vatistas, N.J., J.R. Snyder, G. Carlson, B. Johnson, R.M. Arthur, M. Thurmond, H. Zhou and K.L. Lloyd, 1999b. Cross-sectional study of gastric ulcers of the squamous mucosa in thoroughbred racehorses. Equine Vet J Suppl. 29: 34-39.

White, G., S.R. McClure, R. Sifferman, J.E. Holste, C. Fleishman, M.J. Murray and L.G. Cramer, 2007. Effects of short-term light to heavy exercise on gastric ulcer development in horses and efficacy of omeprazole paste in preventing gastric ulceration. J Am Vet Med Assoc 230: 1680-1682.

White, N.A., 2006. Equine Colic: VI Prognosis and Prevention. Proc AAEP Ann Conv 52: 169-173.

White, S.L., 1998. Fluid, electrolyte, and acid-base balances in three-day, combined-training horses. Vet Clin North Am Equine Pract 14: 137-145.

Widenhouse, T.V., G.G. Lester and A.M. Merritt, 2002. Effect of hydrochloric acid, pepsin, or taurocholate on bioelectric properties of gastric squamous mucosa in horses. Am J Vet Res. 63: 744-749.

Williamson, K.K., M.D. Willard, E.C. McKenzie, C.M. Royer, M.E. Payton and M.S. Davis, 2007. Efficacy of famotidine for the prevention of exercise-induced gastritis in racing Alaskan sled dogs. J Vet Intern Med. 21: 924-927.

Williamson, L. and M. Barton, 1996. Endotoxemia in 3 day event horses. Proc Equine Exer Physiol Res Meet 12. cited by Barton *et al.* (2003).

Wilson, D.E., 1991. Role of prostaglandins in gastroduodenal mucosal protection. J Clin Gastroenterol.13 Suppl 1: S65-71.

Woie, L., B. Kaada, and P.K. Opstad, 1986. Increase in plasma vasoactive intestinal polypeptide (VIP) in muscular exercise in humans. Gen Pharmacol. 17: 321-326.

Zeyner, A., H. Kirbach and M. Furll, 2002. Effects of substituting starch with fat on the acid-base and mineral status of female horses. Equine Vet J Suppl, 85-91.

Zhang, W., W.L. Frankel, A. Bain, D. Choi, D.M. Klurfeld and J.L. Rombeau, 1995. Glutamine reduces bacterial translocation after small bowel transplantation in cyclosporine-treated rats. J Surg Res. 58: 159-164.

Sudden poor performance in the equine athlete: could it be the heart?

Lesley Young[1] and Gunther van Loon[2]
[1]Moat End, Dunstall Green Road, CB8 8TZ Ousden, Suffolk, United Kingdom; lesleyeyoung@googlemail.com
[2]Department Internal Diseases of Large Animals, Faculty Veterinary Medicine, University Gent, Salisburylaan 133, 9820 Merelbeke, Belgium; Gunther.vanloon@rug.ac.be

General

As the readers are well aware, the main causes of poor performance in horses are lack of ability and inappropriate training. Only once respiratory and orthopaedic diseases have been ruled as a cause of sudden catastrophic loss of form, should attention be focused on the cardiovascular system. Cardiovascular causes of poor performance are fairly infrequent, although many horses have cardiovascular dysfunction, especially cardiac murmurs, and as a consequence the significance of cardiac abnormalities can be difficult to determine in individuals and care must be taken not to over-interpret them. Not uncommonly, the heart is often blamed for loss of performance when completely innocent and, conversely, on the rare occasion cardiac disease is significant, it is not uncommon for it to be totally overlooked. This presentation will attempt to introduce some perspective into investigating the cardiovascular abnormalities most likely to adversely effect performance in the equine athlete. The presentation will use case studies to illustrate the approach to these cases and to illustrate the typical presentations of performance limiting cardiac disease.

Approach to suspected cardiac dysfunction

- Take accurate performance history
- Review previous medical history: were murmurs present previously?
- Careful cardiac auscultation at rest. Establish cardiac rate and rhythm and diagnose any cardiac murmurs
- Perform an exercising ECG during appropriate exercise: is heart rate and rhythm normal? In case of sustained atrial fibrillation: are there any ventricular arrhythmias as well?
- Echocardiography: may be indicated, esp. in case of significant murmurs
- Haematology and biochemistry if paroxysmal AF is suspected or in case VPCs or VT is found.

How to take and exercising EKG

The technique of taking a resting electrocardiogram (EKG) using a base-apex lead configuration is now well established in equine practice; most equine practices being equipped with both the expertise and the technology to perform the task. Whilst the method can be valuable in confirming a diagnosis of sustained arrhythmias, like atrial fibrillation, or to diagnose the origin of premature beats, a resting EKG usually offers little to the client in establishing a prognosis for future use of their horse.

The limitations of a resting EKG arise largely because of the enormous cardiac reserve of the horse which means that performance limiting cardiac disease, or abnormal rhythms during exercise, rarely manifest themselves at rest. This is confounded by the fact that alterations in resting cardiac rhythm are common in athletic horses because of normal high parasympathetic drive, yet some of these rhythms can also occur as a result of cardiac pathology. As a result, the effect of a resting arrhythmia on performance, or the effect of exercise on an arrhythmia, can only be established, if an EKG can be taken during strenuous exercise when sympathetic tone and myocardial oxygen demand are increased and parasympathetic influence is reduced.

In the past exercising EKG examination, though well described in the equine literature, was restricted to the specialist cardiologist, or the performance laboratory; largely due very high cost of radiotelemetric EKG equipment. However the newest technology, based on palm top and lap top computers, or specialized battery-operated devices, has become increasingly affordable for equine veterinarians in Europe. As a result it is timely to review the methodology and potential applications of the new generation of EKG devices capable of producing high quality exercising electrocardiographs in performance horses.

Methodology

The use of limb leads for recording EKG traces is not appropriate during exercise: wires and electrodes attached to the limbs are poorly tolerated, even at rest and movement artefact during exercise renders them entirely useless. Crocodile clips to make electrical contact with the skin are also contraindicated for similar reasons. In any event, limb leads, have no practical purpose in equids because the pattern of depolarization of the equine ventricle precludes using multiple vectors to assess cardiac size and mean electrical axis, so there is no point using anything other than a simple positive-negative lead system to record cardiac rhythm. As a result the base apex-lead in which single electrodes are placed above and below the heart is used for all equine EKG recordings, as this lead system produces large complexes, which are easy to identify.

The conventional base apex lead placement in which the positive electrode is placed on the sternum and the negative electrode on the right jugular furrow is modified slightly for exercising recordings to reduce movement artefact caused by neck flexion and extension during movement. This more vertical modification of the familiar system still produces large 'QRS' deflections, but the atrial deflection (P wave) is slightly smaller in amplitude than that of a true base-apex configuration. Nevertheless the P wave will still be clearly visible during exercise.

Figure 1 shows placement of 4 silver/silver chloride adhesive electrodes that is suitable for recording an electrocardiogram during ridden exercise. For four lead systems as in this case, the positive, left arm electrode (usually green) is positioned near to the left cardiac apex, and the negative electrode, right arm (usually red) is placed on the left shoulder area. The third Einthoven lead, the left leg (usually yellow) is also placed caudal to the cardiac apex. This allows 2 identical tracings to be obtained from lead 1 and lead 2 in the Einthoven 3 lead system, allowing for a 'spare', should one of the ventral leads be displaced. The trace in Lead 3 which is recorded between the left arm and left leg will be of no diagnostic value, due to the close apposition of these electrodes at the cardiac apex, but a rhythm trace only is required from a horse, so this is not a serious limitation. The fourth earth electrode, when present (usually black) is then attached on the shoulder close to the negative, right arm electrode.

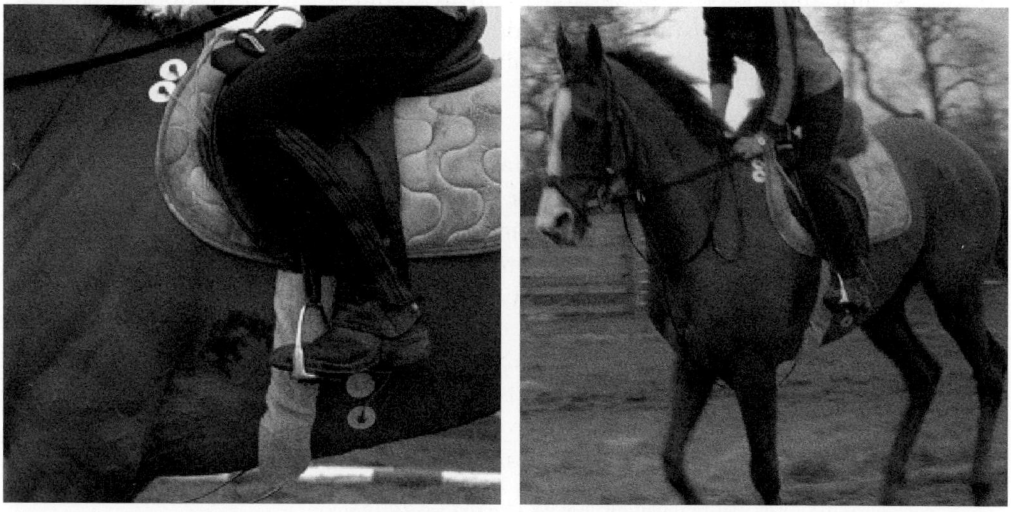

Figure 1. Configuration of electrodes to record an EKG during ridden exercise.

The precise positioning of the electrodes is unimportant provided that the positive is below and slightly caudal to the heart, and negative above and slightly cranial to it. Ideally the electrodes should remain visible to the rider and/or the examiner, so that they can be reattached easily, should they become dislodged. A position where they are least likely to be affected by the saddle or girth slipping backwards, or by the rider's hands or legs is obviously ideal. The recording device can be attached to the metal 'd' ring just below the pommel of most saddles. For harness racing, the electrodes must be similarly positioned away from any moving harness straps. The precise location of particularly the ventral electrodes or the device must often be varied slightly depending on the style of tack, or rider's leg position.

EKG equipment

Traditionally, radiotelelemetric or digital Holter[1] recording systems were used to obtain exercising traces. The former units use a local transmitter carried by the horse that continuously radio transmits the EKG signal to a local recorder. These units are expensive and also require that the recorder remain within at least 250 m of the exercising horse. This can create practical problems for many equine athletes, unless the horse regularly exercises with a scurry or there is good vehicular access to the exercise grounds.

Digital Holter monitors are also effective, but can be expensive unless they can also be used for other applications such as 24-hour EKG recordings in a small animal environment. These devices require specialised software for reading and interpretation of the stored EKG data, although data can be acquired for days at a time and is especially valuable for investigating horses with sporadic collapse. Commercial companies or individuals will read these recordings on a per case basis, reducing the practice's capital outlay, but such providers are generally more familiar with small animal traces.

The newest technology used to obtain these data is based on personal computers and a digital data logger[2]. These units are the most widely applicable and affordable for equine practitioners in a field environment. Importantly, for general practitioners who might be unfamiliar with interpretation of EKG recordings during exercise, the digital format of the data allows them to be emailed easily to specialists for review.

[1] Lifecard CF, Del Mar Reynolds Medical Inc 13 Irvine CA 92618 USA

[2] Televet 100, Kruuse, Denmark

Cardiovascular causes of poor performance

Dysrhythmias

Dysrhythmias occur commonly in resting horses and with the notable exception of atrial fibrillation (AF), usually do not affect performance.

Atrial Fibrillation

This dysrhythmia is the commonest cardiovascular cause of poor performance in horses. The approximate incidence of the sustained form of the dysrhythmia is 1% in National Hunt Thoroughbreds in the UK with prevalence increasing to almost 3% in the older mixed population. When present, it always affects performance in racehorses and high level three-day eventers. The prevalence of the sustained form of AF is lower in flat racing Thoroughbreds and smaller horses, but it is likely that paroxysmal AF occurs more commonly than we appreciate in all horses. At rest, when diastole is long and cardiac output is low, the loss of the atrial contraction has little effect. However during exercise, when diastole is short, peak cardiac output is reduced by the lack of atrial contraction. In addition, the increased sympathetic tone allows too many atrial impulses to conduct to the ventricles, resulting in a disproportionate tachycardia, which further reduces cardiac function. The performance history of these horses reflects compromise at maximum effort. Depending on the training regime, the problem may not be apparent at home. If fibrillation occurs suddenly during a race, the horse may pull up in extreme distress, recovering after a few minutes. In hunters, performance problems are seen during intense exercise usually up hills. Signs of poor performance are generally less obvious in dressage horses, show jumpers and hacks despite the presence of sustained AF.

On the EKG, atrial fibrillation is characterized by the absence of P waves, presence of f waves, normal QRS morphology but irregularly irregular RR intervals (Figure 2).

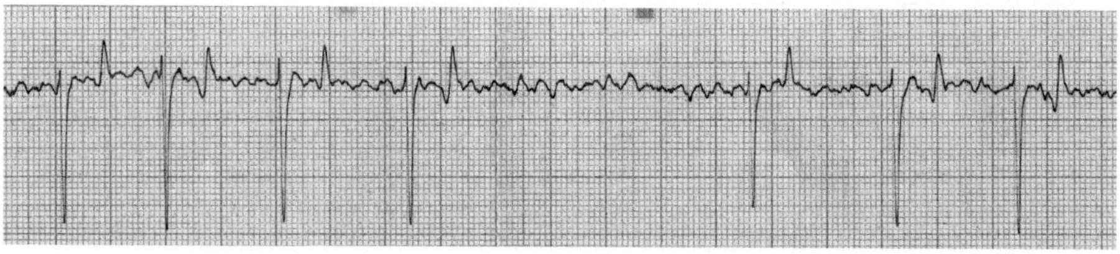

Figure 2. Electrocardiogram recorded at a paper speed of 25 mm/sec. Baseline undulations ('f' waves), total absence of 'p' waves and irregular irregularity of 'qrs' complexes are characteristic of sustained atrial fibrillation.

Atrial fibrillation can present in isolation ('lone' atrial fibrillation) or secondary to atrial enlargement (e.g. as a results of mitral regurgitation) and heart failure. Ultrasonographic examination should be used to select the lone fibrillators because successful treatment of atrial fibrillation should result in return to previous exercise tolerance. Successful treatment can be achieved with oral quinidine sulphate or transvenous electrical cardioversion. After cardioversion, no further medical treatment is given. The advised resting period after cardioversion varies from a few days (acute fibrillation) to two months (chronic fibrillation of more than 4 months) for the atria to fully recover. Horses with significant predisposing cardiac disease are generally not treated because of the lower success rate and the higher recurrence rate. In some horses, recurrence of paroxysmal or sustained atrial fibrillation is a problem, although some owners and trainers become aware of the trigger factors and learn to manage them accordingly. In other cases when frequent recurrence or poor tolerance of treatment occurs, an alternative career can often be found for the horse. Horses in which cardioversion fails or in which the dysrhythmia is not affecting performance, and in which the exercise EKG does not indicate other abnormalities than atrial fibrillation, can also be used for less demanding exercise.

Murmurs

Mitral and tricuspid valve regurgitation

Murmurs are extremely common in horses (Table 1) however they rarely affect performance. In a recent survey by Karen Blissitt of the RDSVS of the owners of 109 horses with non functional cardiac murmurs, 73 owners (67%) thought the murmur did not affect their horses performance, whereas 8 (7.3%), felt performance was affected by the murmur.

Further evidence of a lack of effect of compensated valve dysfunction in UK racehorses was provided by a large epidemiological study of 586 race fit horses. These data also showed that neither regurgitation assessed by colour flow Doppler, nor murmurs assessed by auscultation were negatively associated with Timeform rating, an index of UK racehorse quality, in any of the groups of racehorses studied.

Although uncommon, severe AV valve disease that has progressed to cause heart failure is always associated with poor performance. Most commonly such failure is associated with catastrophic mitral regurgitation often in conjunction with secondary atrial fibrillation. Progression of mitral or tricuspid valve disease to cause cardiac failure is rare. To differentiate between compensated and decompensated disease, check resting heart rate and look for the presence of a widely radiating murmur associated with a palpable precordial thrill.

Table 1. Prevalence proportions (95% confidence intervals) of murmurs and regurgitation at the mitral, tricuspid and aortic valves in horses of different race types, derived from the first observations taken from every horse (n= 586).

%	Type of horse						Statistical significance*
	2 yr olds	Sprints, >2 yr olds	Longer races, >2 yr olds	Bumpers	Hurdlers	Steeplechasers	
Tricuspid Valve							
All murmurs	20 (12-28)	27 (11-42)	24 (13-34)	40 (32-48)	46 (40-52)	44 (38-51)	<0.0001
Murmurs graded ≥3/6	7 (2-12)	7 (0-16)	12 (4-19)	11 (6-16)	14 (10-18)	15 (10-19)	0.4
All regurgitation	75 (66-83)	87 (75-99)	89 (82-97)	81 (75-87)	86 (82-90)	89 (85-93)	0.02
Regurgitation scored ≥6/9	1 (0-3)	7 (0-16)	9 (2-16)	8 (4-12)	10 (7-14)	13 (8-17)	0.1
Mitral Valve							
All murmurs	7 (2-12)	10 (0-21)	18 (9-27)	13 (8-19)	19 (14-23)	23 (18-29)	0.008
Murmurs graded ≥3/6	1 (0-3)	3 (0-10)	3 (0-7)	1 (0-2)	1 (0-2)	3 (1-6)	0.2
All regurgitation	29 (20-38)	53 (35-71)	60 (48-72)	40 (33-48)	46 (41-52)	52 (45-58)	0.001
Regurgitation scored ≥6/9	1 (0-3)	3 (0-10)	2 (0-5)	2 (0-4)	3 (1-5)	6 (3-9)	0.2
Aortic Valve							
All murmurs	1 (0-3)	0 (0-0)	0 (0-0)	3 (0-5)	4 (1-6)	7 (3-10)	0.1
Murmurs graded ≥3/6	0 (0-0)	0 (0-0)	0 (0-0)	1 (0-2)	0 (0-1)	2 (0-4)	0.2
All regurgitation	38 (29-48)	57 (39-74)	54 (42-66)	54 (46-62)	57 (52-63)	65 (59-71)	0.1
Regurgitation scored ≥6/9	0 (0-0)	0 (0-0)	0 (0-0)	3 (0-5)	3 (1-5)	5 (2-8)	0.3
Any murmur or regurgitation	84 (77-91)	90 (79-100)	90 (82-97)	94 (90-98)	94 (92-97)	97 (94-99)	0.003

* Likelihood ratio statistic derived from univariable logistic regression models

From Young *et al.*, 2008.

Murmur assessed by auscultation (1 -6 scale); Regurgitation assessed by colour flow Doppler (1 – 9 scale)

Aortic insufficiency

Aortic insufficiency is most commonly detected in middle aged to older horses and is the least common of the murmurs encountered in race and sports horse practice. The condition is progressive and is associated with thickening and fibrosis of the valve leaflets. It is usually initially detected as a low-grade murmur (grade 1-2/6) in horses over 10 years of age, and then progresses very slowly. In older horses, it rarely affects performance, as progression occurs over many years and work expectations usually decrease with age. Aortic insufficiency causes volume overload of the left ventricle resulting in dilatation. Pleasure horses can continue to perform adequately even with severe aortic insufficiency and marked volume overload. However a dilated ventricle works against increased afterload and has an increased oxygen requirement. In aortic insufficiency, there is decreased coronary perfusion due to reduced diastolic aortic pressure and oxygen delivery to the myocardium is compromised. Increased oxygen demand and reduced coronary reserve increases susceptibility to ventricular arrhythmias that can result in sudden death. Affected horses must be monitored regularly so they can be retired from work before severe ventricular dilatation develops.

Aortic insufficiency also occurs sporadically in younger horses. The condition may be associated with the presence of a small ventricular septal defect or there may be no obvious pathology other than valve leaflet prolapse ±dilatation of the aortic root. Severe aortic insufficiency in such animals can progress to heart failure, although in some cases progression is very slow and the racing career is not noticeably compromised. Progression of this condition is impossible to predict in individuals, so all affected cases should be carefully monitored.

Ventricular septal defect

The size of a ventricular septal defect will determine its effects on performance. If the defect is small and restricts blood flow between the two ventricles, performance will not be affected. If however the defect is large, horses perform below their genetic potential. The intensity of the expected exercise will also influence whether performance decrements are observed. Show and pleasure horses perform with relatively large ventricular septal defects that would probably be incompatible with a successful racing career. Echocardiography is valuable for determining the likely significance of a ventricular septal defect. Murmur loudness is not necessarily associated with a poor prognosis

Vascular causes

Aortoiliac thromboembolism

This is an occasional cause of reduced performance in horses. It appears to be more common in male horses and can occur in any age group. Symptoms vary from mild hind limb stiffness that reduces performance to more severe unilateral or bilateral hindlimb lameness. Although one would generally expect to recognise the characteristic clinical signs associated with this condition, this is not invariably the case, and we have diagnosed this disorder in horses referred for poor performance investigation with no previous history of exercise-induced lameness.

Less common cardiac causes of diminished performance

Bradydysrhythmias

In the resting horse many bradydysrhythmias are of no clinical significance, as within limits, cardiac output can be maintained by an increase in stroke volume. The trained horse has an increased resting stroke volume and therefore the resting heart rate is normally low. During exercise however, there is an increased requirement for muscle perfusion and cardiac output must increase to maintain arterial blood pressure and blood flow. The major part of this increase in cardiac output is caused by an increase in heart rate. Therefore if a low heart rate is maintained during exercise, cardiac output will be inadequate and performance will be limited. Occasionally these conditions are associated with collapse at rest and during exercise. Examples include 3rd degree AV block and advanced 2nd degree AV block. Pathological sinus bradycardia is found most commonly in elderly ponies and donkeys. Occasionally horses affected with profound 2nd degree AV block and sinus bradycardia respond favourably to daily oral administration of β_2 adrenoreceptor agonist drugs e.g. clenbuterol. In general for bradydysrhythmias, the prognosis is guarded to poor.

Tachydysrhythmias

Tachydysrhythmias reduce cardiac output by reducing the time available for ventricular filling. In addition ventricular depolarisations reduce cardiac output further by decreasing stroke volume due to uncoordinated contractions.

Atrial premature systoles

Atrial premature systoles are detected fairly frequently in horses in training and affect performance only if they produce excessive heart rates during exercise, or when they predispose to paroxysmal atrial fibrillation. More commonly the premature excitatory focus is over-ridden as sinus nodal rate increases, and the extrasystoles disappear, thus poor performance is not usually a feature.

Figure 3a presents a resting EKG (25 mm/s 10 mm/mV) that was obtained from a 13 year-old cob after an abnormal rhythm was noted during auscultation. The horse was otherwise asymptomatic. There are multiple atrial premature beats (arrowed) present at rest.

Figure 3b presents a second trace coming from the same horse during canter (heart rate 169 beats per minute) and illustrates why per se atrial premature beats are rarely associated with poor performance. The rhythm is now entirely regular, as the sinus node rate has now overridden the ectopic focus. The ectopic beats only returned some 15 minutes after the horse returned to his stable and his rate fell to below 60 beats per minute.

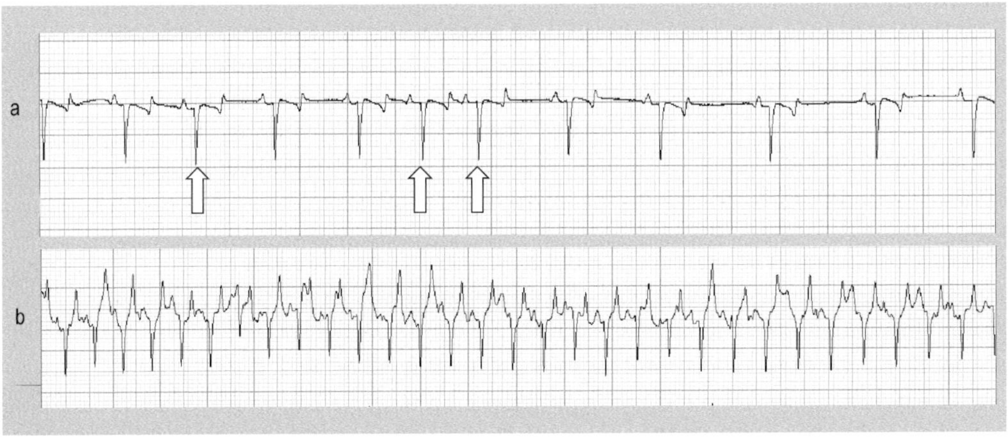

Figure 3a. Resting EKG (25 mm/s 10 mm/mV) that was obtained from a 13 year-old cob after an abnormal rhythm was noted during auscultation. The horse was otherwise asymptomatic. There are multiple atrial premature beats (arrowed) present at rest.
Figure 3b. Second trace coming from the same horse during canter (heart rate 169 beats per minute) and illustrates why per se atrial premature beats are rarely associated with poor performance. The rhythm is now entirely regular, as the sinus node rate has now overridden the ectopic focus. The ectopic beats only returned some 15 minutes after the horse returned to his stable and his rate fell to below 60 beats per minute.

Ventricular premature systoles

Ventricular premature systoles may be caused by electrolyte disorders, myocardial inflammation or degeneration, intoxication, but in most horses the exact cause remains unclear. Ventricular premature contractions will also affect performance if they produce a tachycardia during exercise. This dysrhythmia is of more concern due to the risk of sustained ventricular tachycardia predisposing to ventricular fibrillation. This situation is likely to be exacerbated during exercise when sympathetic tone increases. Ventricular extrasystoles are very common in normal racehorses during the recovery period after fast exercise, occurring in over 60% of race fit thoroughbreds in 1 treadmill study. They should therefore not be over-interpreted and provide another reason why taking an ECG immediately after exercise is not advisable and no substitute for an exercising ECG.

The example shown in Figure 4 was taken from a 16 year-old Thoroughbred during fast work on an all-weather gallop (10 mm/mV, 25 mm/s). There had been no change in the clinical characteristics of his grade 4/6 diastolic murmur over 3 years. His resting heart rate was 32 beats per minute with regular 2nd degree atrioventricular block.

The trace shows a triplet of ventricular ectopic beats. This triplet occurred at a heart rate of 168 beats per minute during hack canter. Multiple episodes of ventricular and junctional ectopic beats occurred during this exercise session, although the horse appeared clinically normal

Regardless of any effect on performance, as this rhythm is a trigger for ventricular fibrillation, the horse was immediately retired from ridden work.

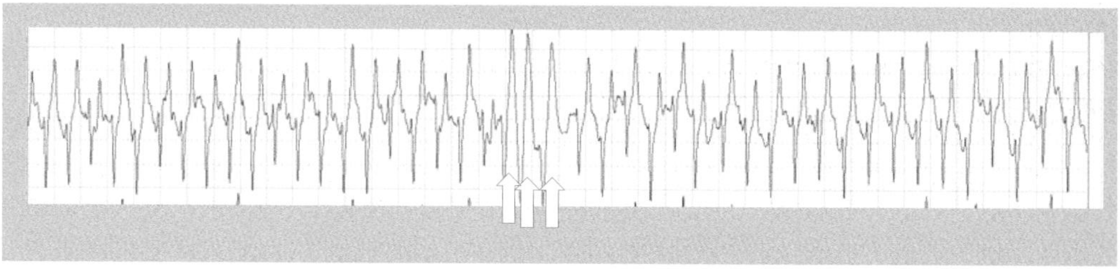

Figure 4. A 16 year-old Thoroughbred during fast work on an all-weather gallop (10 mm/mV, 25 mm/s).

Some useful references

Birks, E.K., M.M. Durando and B.B.J. Martin, 2004. Clinical exercise testing:evaluation of the poor performing athlete. In: K.W. Hinchcliff, A.J. Kaneps and R.J. Goer (Eds.) Equine Sports Medicine and Surgery: Basic and Clinical Sciences of the Equine Athlete, Edinburgh: Saunders, p. 9-19.

Durando, M.M. and L.E. Young, 2003. Cardiovascular examination and diagnostic techniques. In: N.E. Robinson (Eds.) Current Therapy in Equine Medicine, Saunders, Philadelphia, 930 pp.

Hamlin, R.L., W.L. Klepinger, K.W. Gilpin and C.R. Smith, 1972. Autonomic control of heart rate in the horse. Am J Physiol 222: 976-978.

Jose-Cunilleras, E., L.E Young, J.R. Newton and D.J. Martin, 2006. Cardiac arrhythmias during and after treadmill exercise in poorly performing thoroughbred racehorses. Equine Vet J Suppl. 36: 163-170.

Martin, B.B., Jr., V.B. Reef, E.J. Parente and A.D. Sage, 2000. Causes of poor performance of horses during training, racing, or showing: 348 cases (1992-1996). J Am Vet Med Assoc 216: 554-558.

Ohmura, H., A. Hiraga, T. Takahashi, M. Kai and J.H. Jones, 2003. Risk factors for atrial fibrillation during racing in slow-finishing horses. J Am Vet Med Assoc 223: 84-88.

Poole, D.C. and H.H. Erikson, 2004. Heart and Vessels: Function during exercise and response to training. In: K.W. Hinchcliff, A.J. Kaneps and R.J. Goer (Eds.) Equine Sports Medicine and Surgery, Oxford UK: Elsevier Science Limited, p. 699-727.

Ryan, N., C.M. Marr and A.J. McGladdery, 2005. Survey of cardiac arrhythmias during submaximal and maximal exercise in thoroughbred racehorses. Equine Vet J. May 37: 265-268.

Young, L.E., 2003. Diseases of the heart and Vessels. In: K.W. Hinchcliff, A.J. Kaneps and R.J. Goer (Eds.) Equine Sports Medicine and Surgery: Basic and Clinical Sciences of the Equine Athlete, Edinburgh: Saunders, p. 728-769.

Young, L.E., K. Rogers and J.L.N. Wood, 2008. Heart murmurs and valvular regurgitation in Thoroughbred racehorses: Epidemiology and associations with athletic performance Journal of Veterinary Internal Medicine 22: 418-426.

Prevalence and clinical management of equine exertional rhabdomyolysis syndrome in different types of sport horses

José Luis L. Rivero[1] *and Richard J. Piercy*[2]
[1]*Departamento de Anatomía, Facultad de Veterinaria, Universidad de Córdoba, Campus de Rabanales, Edificio de Sanidad Animal, Crtra. Madrid-Cádiz, km 396, 14008 Córdoba, Spain; an1lorij@uco.es*
[2]*Comparative Neuromuscular Diseases Laboratory, Department of Veterinary Clinical Sciences, Royal Veterinary College, Hawkshead Lane, Hertfordshire AL9 7TA, United Kingdom; rpiercy@rvc.ac.uk*

Introduction

Neuromuscular problems have long been recognised as performance-limiting and (or) career-ending disorders in equine athletes. Of these, exertional rhabdomyolysis (henceforth, ER) is the most prevalent (Piercy and Rivero, 2004). Estimates suggest that approximately 5-7% of Thoroughbred racehorses may be affected (Cole *et al.*, 2004; MacLeay *et al.*, 1999a; Upjohn *et al.*, 2005) and the incidence is similar in Standardbred trotters. Other neuromuscular disorders (both myogenic and neurogenic in origin) also affect equine athletes but given their much lower incidence (see Piercy and Rivero, 2004 for a recent review) they are less important to the equine practitioner.

ER consists of a degenerative and regenerative process of the skeletal musculature, generally induced (but usually not caused) by exercise. In the last 15 years, research advances have provided greater insight into this syndrome. Of greatest importance was realisation that ER comprises several myopathies that despite similarities in clinical presentation, differ considerably in regards to pathophysiology (Piercy and Rivero, 2004). In addition, recent work examining effective management of horses with these diseases, particularly regarding diet and exercise, has significantly reduced the severity of ER in many horses (Valberg, 2005).

Clinical signs of ER are highly variable, ranging from subclinical to severe. In the former cases, an underlying muscle problem may be hard to identify in an animal with unexplained poor performance; in the latter, massive muscle necrosis and concomitant myoglobinuria may precede renal failure and occasionally death. The most common clinical signs however include muscle pain on deep palpation of lumbar and / or gluteal regions, muscle tremors, stiffness and occasionally in chronic cases, muscle atrophy. Excessive sweating, tachypnoea and tachycardia are common in moderate-severe acute cases. The clinical (presumptive) diagnosis of ER is based on a thorough assessment of the history and clinical examination, combined with identification of (sometimes massively) increased plasma creatine kinase (CK) and aspartate transferase (AST) activities. Muscle biopsy is helpful in distinguishing various forms of recurrent ER and provides information about the severity of any underlying primary myopathic disorder, hence enabling assessment of prognosis.

There are two clinical forms of ER, sporadic (generally acquired) and intermittent (usually inherited). Horses that experience a single episode or infrequent episodes of muscle necrosis induced by exercise are categorised as having sporadic ER, whereas horses that have repeated episodes of ER, even with only mild exertion, are classified as having intermittent ER. It is difficult to document with certainty the cause of most sporadic forms of ER, however over-training and muscle strain, dietary deficiencies of electrolytes, vitamin E and selenium or excessive exercise in conjunction with herpes or influenza virus infection have all been proposed. The evidence supporting some of these causes is somewhat speculative or unsubstantiated.

Intermittent ER is believed often to be associated with primary inherited (genetic) myopathies. At present, two specific forms of intermittent ER, termed polysaccharide storage myopathy (PSSM) and recurrent exertional rhabdomyolysis (RER), have been recognised in several breeds. A specific cause of RER has been identified in Thoroughbreds (Lentz *et al.*, 1999) due to defective regulation of intracellular calcium. Because definitive muscle contracture testing *in vitro* (Lentz *et al.*, 1999) has not been widely examined, it is unclear whether all Thoroughbreds share this same disorder, or whether horses of other breeds are affected with the same abnormality. As such, most horses without other specific changes on muscle biopsy are regarded as having an idiopathic myopathy.

PSSM was initially described in Quarter horses and horses with Quarter horse bloodlines (Valberg *et al.*, 1992), but a similar disorder has been recognised in many other breeds (Quiroz-Rothe *et al.*, 2002; Valentine and Cooper, 2005; McCue *et al.*, 2006). This is a glycogen storage disorder characterised by the accumulation of glycogen and abnormal polysaccharide complexes in a considerable proportion of skeletal muscle fibres. The metabolic defect involves abnormal regulation of glycogen synthesis rather than a defect in its utilisation, and recently a single base pair missense mutation has been identified in the skeletal muscle glycogen synthase 1 gene of affected horses (McCue *et al.*, 2008). The mutation confers increased activity to the enzyme, thereby likely upsetting the carefully controlled balance between the 2 enzymes responsible for glycogen synthesis (glycogen synthase and branching enzyme). The disorder is autosomal dominant (McCue *et al.*, 2008), hence breeding a horse with this disease results in a 50% chance that the offspring will be affected, regardless of the stallion or mare chosen as a breeding partner. Differential diagnosis of the different intermittent forms of ER is based upon direct genotyping from DNA (hair roots or whole blood) and by the analysis of muscle biopsy samples. Periodic acid Schiff-positive and α–amylase resistant inclusion bodies are a consistent feature of PSSM (Figure 1).

Despite the syndrome's extensive study for over 100 years, particularly in certain racing breeds (Thoroughbreds, Standardbreds, Arabians and Quarter horses), the syndrome has received considerably less attention in other types of sport horses used for high-level competition: for example, in dressage, show-jumping and eventing. There is now sufficient evidence that both the prevalence and presenting complaints of the different specific forms of intermittent ER are breed-specific (McCue *et al.*, 2006). To date, the incidence and clinical pathological features of many European breeds used with sporting purposes (i.e., Spanish purebred –SPB-, saddle horses, Warmbloods, etc.) is practically unknown (Quiroz-Rothe *et al.*, 2002). We present here a retrospective study of demographic data and main clinical features of specific forms of the ER syndrome in different types of athletic horses, with particular focus on objective comparison between breeds mainly used for sporting disciplines (dressage, show-jumping and others) vs. traditional breeds of racehorses used in gallop, trotting and endurance competitions. Data selection is based on a considerable number of clinical cases of horses with suspected neuromuscular disease from which a muscle biopsy had been submitted to the laboratory by referring practitioners across the European Union, seen over several years.

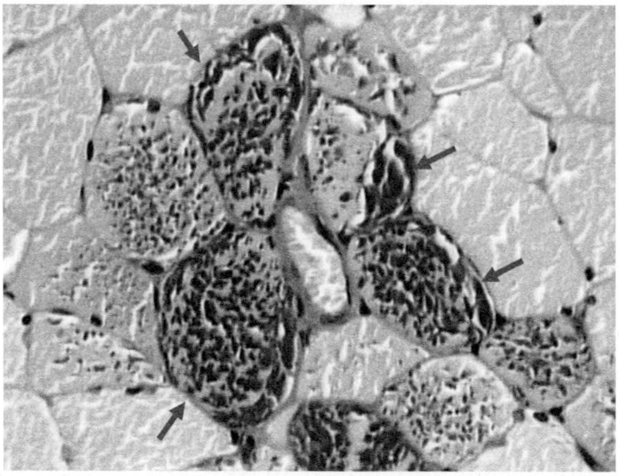

Figure 1. Periodic acid Schiff's stain after amylase digestion of a cross section of semimembranosus muscle from a horse with polysaccharide storage myopathy. Arrows denote muscle fibres with granular abnormal polysaccharide resistant to amylase digestion.

Materials and methods

The study considered retrospectively a total of 369 cases of horses with suspected neuromuscular disorders from which muscle biopsies had been submitted to the Muscular Biopathology Laboratory at the University of Cordoba (Spain) between September 1998 and December 2006. Available data for each case included breed, age, sex, training history, discipline, clinical history, main physical examination findings and (in the majority of cases –314/369, 85.1%) serum CK and AST activities.

Open surgical muscle biopsy samples from the *semimembranosus/semitendinosus* muscles (shipped by referring veterinarians) and samples taken at our veterinary teaching hospital from the *M. gluteus medius* and (or) *M. longissimus lumborum* (Quiroz-Rothe *et al.*, 2002) were examined. Muscle sections were stained with a battery of stains and examined by microscopy for specific types of ER.

The total prevalence of each specific form of ER was calculated by dividing the number of horses with a specific diagnosis of ER by the total number of cases included. The prevalence of each muscular problem within each category (breed, sex, age group, training situation and sport discipline) was obtained by dividing the number of cases affected by each particular muscular problem by the total number of cases included in that specific category. Differences in the prevalence of each specific form of ER as a function of demographic data, natural history and clinical examination findings were calculated using a Pearson's Chi-square analysis, considering significant differences at $P<0.05$.

Results

Of the 369 clinical cases, 262 horses were identified with a specific form of ER based on their clinical history, clinical examination and muscle biopsy histopathology (i.e 70.1% of horses with suspected neuromuscular disorder that underwent a muscle biopsy). Of these, 32 (12.2%) were identified with sporadic ER, 114 with PSSM (43.5%) and 116 (44.3%) with idiopathic exertional myopathy.

The study examined many different breeds that were assigned to four main categories: SPB, sport breeds, racing breeds and other breeds (Table 1). As expected, both the total number of cases and the within breed prevalence of the three specific forms of ER syndrome varied significantly among breeds. This prevalence was significantly lower in SPB horses (81/138, 59%) than in sport (108/130, 83%) and racing (69/83, 83%) breeds. PSSM was the most prevalent form of ER in Quarter horses, SPBs and other sport breeds, whereas the idiopathic forms of ER were commonest in Standardbreds, Thoroughbreds and Arabians (Figure 2).

Table 1. Demographic data of horses considered in the study.

Breed	Submissions	Sex		Age			Training	
		Male	Female	x±sem	Range		In	Out
SPB	138 (37.4)	108 (78.3)	30 (21.7)	5.3±0.2	0.5-16	Aa	83 (60.1)	55 (39.9)
Sport breeds	130 (35.2)	91 (70.0)	39 (30.0)	8.0±0.3	4-18	C	112 (86.2)	18 (13.9)
Warmblood	61 (16.5)	40 (65.6)	21 (34.4)	8.1±0.3	5-12	b	53 (86.9)	8 (13.1)
Anglo-arab	58 (15.7)	45 (77.6)	13 (22.4)	7.8±0.5	4-18	bc	48 (82.8)	10 (17.2)
Saddle breeds	11 (3.0)	6 (54.6)	5 (45.5)	8.7±0.5	6-10	bd	11 (100)	
Racing breeds	83 (22.5)	37 (44.6)	46 (55.4)	6.6±0.3	0.8-12	B	65 (78.3)	18 (21.7)
Arab	24 (6.5)	16 (66.7)	8 (33.3)	8.1±0.6	2-12	bc	19 (79.2)	5 (20.8)
Thoroughbred	23 (6.2)	16 (69.6)	7 (30.4)	5.4±0.7	0.8-11	ac	14 (60.9)	9 (39.1)
Standardbred	22 (6.0)		22 (100)	5.8±0.3	4-8	acd	20 (90.9)	2 (9.1)
Quarter horse	14 (3.8)	5 (35.7)	9 (64.3)	6.9±0.8	3-12	ad	12 (85.7)	2 (14.3)
Other breeds	18 (4.9)	12 (66.7)	6 (33.3)	7.1±0.2	5-8	BC	8 (44.4)	10 (55.6)
Ponies	17 (4.6)	11 (64.7)	6 (35.3)	7.1±0.2	5-8	ad	8 (47.1)	9 (52.9)
Draught breeds	1 (0.3)	1 (100)		7.0				1 (100)
Total	369 (100)	248 (67.2)	121 (32.8)	6.7±0.2	10.5-8		268 (72.6)	101 (27.4)

Data are presented as absolute and relative (in brackets) frequencies. For age, descriptive statistics (mean±sem and range) are presented for each breed or breed category; mean values with different letters (either capital or lower case) are statistically different ($P<0.05$). SPB, Spanish pure-breed.

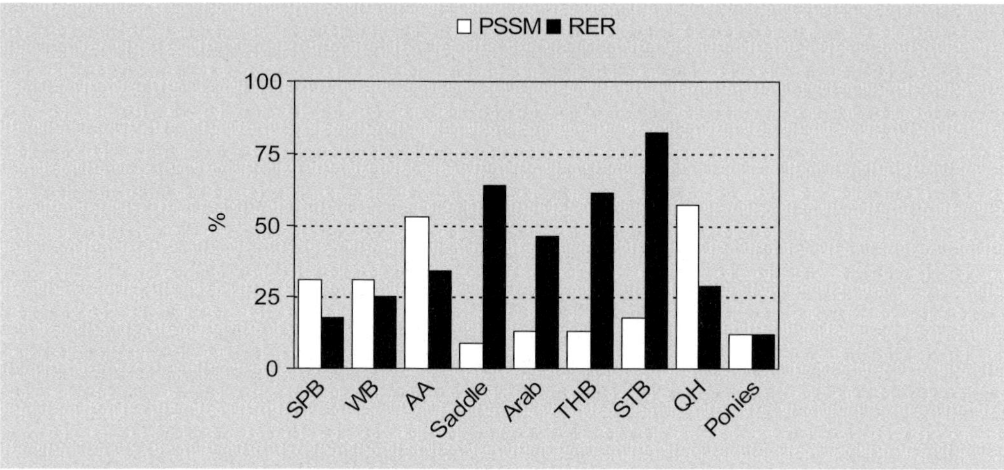

Figure 2. Within breed prevalence of polysaccharide storage myopathy (PSSM) and recurrent exertional rhabdomyolysis (RER). SPB, Spanish purebred; WB, Warmblood; AA, Anglo-arab; THB, Thoroughbred; STB, Standardbred; QH, Quarter horse.

In general, the mean age of horses with ER was significantly lower in SPB horses than in the other breed categories, particularly in males, however this difference reflected the signalment of all submissions to the laboratory within this category and was not specific for ER. The prevalence of ER did not vary significantly between sexes, but the number of cases of PSSM was significantly higher in males (34.7%) than in females (23.1%), the contrary being true for RER (males, 25.2%; females, 42.1%).

Overall, ER syndrome occurred more commonly (215/268, 80.2%) in horses currently in training rather than out (47/101, 46.5%) of training. In addition, the number of cases of ER was significantly higher in sports horses (150/186, 80.7%) and racing breeds (52/58, 89.7%) than in horses with other non-athletic uses (60/125, 48%).

Nearly all cases of ER (254/262, 97%) were associated with recent exercise. The total number of intermittent cases with a length of more than two weeks from onset of clinical signs (194/262, 74%), and the number of cases with recurrent episodes of rhabdomyolysis (224/262, 85.5%) were much more common than the number of acute cases (68/262, 26%) and cases with sporadic clinical presentations (38/262, 14.5%).

In all breeds and for the three specific forms of the ER syndrome, there was pain on palpation of either gluteal or lumbar musculature or both in the vast majority of cases (92%), a clinical finding always present in racing breeds. Muscle atrophy, either uni- or bilateral, of gluteal and / or lumbar musculature was a common clinical feature of intermittent ER, affecting 61% of SPB, 44% sport breeds; however only 16% of racing breeds had this sign.

The presence and severity of muscular signs characteristic of rhabdomyolysis were scored for each clinical case as Grade 0 (absent or asymptomatic), Grade 1 (moderate; e.g., muscle tone abnormalities and/or fasciculation), and Grade 2 (severe; e.g., muscle tremors, muscle cramps, myotonia, spasticity and/or myoglobinuria). In general, asymptomatic (Grade 0) or moderate (Grade 1) cases of rhabdomyolysis were more common in SPB and sport breeds than in racehorses. The number of cases with severe signs (Grade 2) was, however, higher in racehorses than in sport horses. Each clinical ER case was additionally scored according to the extent of gait abnormality ranging from Grade 0 (without gait disturbances), Grade 1 (stiffness, weakness and shortening of the stride in the hind limbs) or Grade 2 (reluctance or refusal to move and/or evidence of clinical lameness). The number of clinical cases of ER with gait abnormalities of either Grade 0 or Grade 1 were more prevalent in racing breeds than in sports horses, whereas gait disturbances of Grade 2 were proportionally more frequent in SPB and sport breeds than in racehorses.

CK and AST activities were also available for most submissions. Clinical cases of ER were classified into three semi-quantitative categories according to their enzymatic activities: Grade 0 (values in the reference range: CK 50-200 UI/L; AST 200-400 UI/L), Grade 1 (moderate increments: CK 200-1000 UI/L; AST 400-1200 UI/L) and Grade 2 (intense increments: CK >1000 UI/L; AST >1200 UI/L). The total number of cases with normal baseline CK and AST activities (Grade 0) was significantly higher in SPB and sport breeds than in racing breeds. However more racing breeds had the highest (Grade 2) category than sports breeds.

Discussion

This data suggests that the prevalence of the ER syndrome is similar in sports horses and in racing breeds, although we cannot rule out the possibility that muscle biopsy submissions may not accurately reflect the actual prevalence of the condition in the general equine population. It did appear however that ER is less of a problem in SPB horses than in the other sports breeds included in the study. Amongst these conditions, a common specific form of this syndrome in sports breeds, including SPB, is PSSM and in the future it will be especially interesting to determine how many of these horses carry the glycogen synthase mutation reported by McCue *et al.* (2008). SPB horses with ER syndrome are, on average, younger than horses belonging to other breeds; the apparent sex bias may reflect a bias within the general population, although a similar increased incidence in females for ER in Thoroughbreds has previously been reported (MacLeay *et al.*, 1999a).

Similar to findings in other breeds, (Valberg *et al.*, 1999; Valberg, 2005), specific forms of intermittent ER (i.e., PSSM and RER) in sport breeds cannot readily be distinguished upon the basis of their clinical signs. Clinical features of the ER syndrome in SPBs are qualitatively and quantitatively similar to those observed in other breeds of sport horses, but different to those commonly recorded in several racing breeds. Unlike other breeds, muscle atrophy in chronic cases of ER is a distinctive clinical feature of the syndrome in SPBs. In general, typical clinical signs of ER and elevated CK and AST activities tended to be more moderate in breeds of sport horses than in racehorses. However evidence of muscle atrophy together with severe gait abnormalities was comparatively more frequent in sport horses than in racehorses.

Practically, this report provides support for considering primary myopathies in horses, especially young adult sport horses, that present with unexplained poor performance, even when classic clinical signs of muscle disease (for example stiffness), are absent. Muscle enzyme activities may only be mildly-moderately elevated, and on occasion, may be within the normal range. Other signs that may support an underlying myopathy include muscle atrophy and gait abnormalities.

Accurate specific diagnosis of the various forms of the ER syndrome is important to rationalise the therapeutic and prophylactic management of each particular case. Although in this study we did not evaluate response to treatments or prophylaxis these are well established. Evidence supports use of oral dantrolene sodium as a prophylactic agent for managing Thoroughbreds with recurrent ER (Edwards *et al.*, 2003; McKenzie *et al.*, 2004): whether the same strategy applies to other breeds with idiopathic ER is uncertain, however in our opinion it is a reasonable option. Although there is controversy over whether the drug should be administered to horses that have had feed withheld overnight, many trainers administer oral dantrolene at 1-2.5 mg/kg approximately 90 minutes before exercise, where it is often used daily, particularly when a horse has been rested, or when the amount of exercise is increasing. There is also good evidence supporting changing the diet for Thoroughbreds with RER: in particular increasing the proportion of calorific intake from fat as opposed to carbohydrate (MacLeay *et al.*, 1999b; McKenzie *et al.*, 2003), although in racehorses this is often hard to achieve. For management of PSSM, it also appears that a high fat, low carbohydrate diet is beneficial (Firshman *et al.*, 2003; Ribeiro *et al.*, 2004; Valberg and Mickelson, 2007). Finally, in both PSSM and RER there is good subjective evidence that horses respond well to regular daily (7 days per week exercise), including the day following racing or strenuous exercise (Valberg and Mickelson, 2007).

In summary, ER is an important cause of poor performance. Within this syndrome are several specific entities that can now be better classified. In combination with genetic testing, muscle biopsy offers a straight forward technique to better characterise these conditions in a variety of breeds.

References

Cole, F.L., D.J. Mellor, D.R. Hodgson and S.W. Reid, 2004. Prevalence and demographic characteristics of exertional rhabdomyolysis in horses in Australia. Vet Rec 155: 625-630.

Edwards, J.G., J.R. Newtont, P.H. Ramzan, R.C. Pilsworth and M.C. Shepherd, 2003. The efficacy of dantrolene sodium in controlling exertional rhabdomyolysis in the Thoroughbred racehorse. Equine Vet J 35: 707-711.

Firshman, A.M., S.J. Valberg, J.B. Bender and C.J. Finno, 2003. Epidemiologic characteristics and management of polysaccharide storage myopathy in Quarter Horses. Am J Vet Res 64: 1319-1327.

Lentz, L.R., S.J. Valberg, L. Herold, G.W. Onan, J.R. Mickelson and E.M. Gallant, 2002. Myoplasmic calcium regulation in myotubes from horses with recurrent exertional rhabdomyolysis. Am J Vet Res 63: 1724-1731.

MacLeay, J.M., S.A. Sorum, S.J. Valberg, W.E. Marsh and M.D. Sorum, 1999a. Epidemiologic analysis of factors influencing exertional rhabdomyolysis in Thoroughbreds. Am J Vet Res 60: 1562-1566.

MacLeay, J.M., S.J. Valberg, J.D. Pagan, F. de laCorte, J. Roberts, J. Billstrom, J. McGinnity and H. Kaese, 1999b. Effect of diet on thoroughbred horses with recurrent exertional rhabdomyolysis performing a standardised exercise test. Equine Vet J Suppl 30: 458-462.

McCue, M.E., W.P. Ribeiro and S.J. Valberg, 2006. Prevalence of polysaccharide storage myopathy in horses with neuromuscular disorders. Equine Vet. J. Suppl 36: 340-344.

McCue, M.E., S.J. Valberg, M.B. Miller, C. Wade, S. DiMauro, H.O. Akman and J.R. Mickelson, 2008. Glycogen synthase (GYS1) mutation causes a novel skeletal muscle glycogenosis. Genomics 91: 458-466.

McKenzie, E.C., S.J. Valberg, S.M. Godden, C.J. Finno and M.J. Murphy, 2004. Effect of oral administration of dantrolene sodium on serum creatine kinase activity after exercise in horses with recurrent exertional rhabdomyolysis. Am J Vet Res 65: 74-79.

McKenzie, E.C., S.J. Valberg, S.M. Godden, J.D. Pagan, J.M. MacLeay, R.J. Geor and G.P. Carlson, 2003. Effect of dietary starch, fat, and bicarbonate content on exercise responses and serum creatine kinase activity in equine recurrent exertional rhabdomyolysis. J Vet Intern Med 17: 693-701.

Piercy, R.J. and J.L.L. Rivero, 2004. Muscle disorders of equine athletes. In: K.W. Hinchcliff, A.J. Kaneps and R.J. Geor (Eds.) Equine sports medicine and surgery, Saunders Elservier, Edingurgh, pp 77-110.

Quiroz-Rothe, E., M. Novales, E. Aguilera-Tejero and J.L.L. Rivero, 2002. Polysaccharidae storage myopathy in the M. longissimus lumborum of showjumpers and dressage horses with back pain. Equine Vet. J. 34: 171-176.

Ribeiro, W.P., S.J. Valberg, J.D. Pagan and B.E. Gustavsson, 2004. The effect of varying dietary starch and fat content on serum creatine kinase activity and substrate availability in equine polysaccharide storage myopathy. J Vet Intern Med 18: 887-894.

Upjohn, M.M., R.M. Archer, R.M. Christley and C.M. McGowan, 2005. Incidence and risk factors associated with exertional rhabdomyolysis syndrome in National Hunt racehorses in Great Britain. Vet Rec 156: 763-766.

Valberg, S.J., 2005. Differential diagnosis and nutritional management of equine exertional rhabdomyolysis. In: A Lindner (Ed.) Applied equine nutrition, Equine Nutrition Conference 2005, Wageningen Academic Publishers, Wageningen, the Netherlands, pp. 139-157.

Valberg, S.F. and J.R. Mickelson, 2007. The interplay of genetics, exercise, and nutrition in polysaccharide storage myopathy. In: ACVIM, Seattle, Washington, USA.

Valberg, S.J., J.R. Mickelson, E.M. Gallant, J.M. MacLeay, L. Lentz, F.D. De La Corte, 1999. Exertional rhabdomyolysis in Quarter Horses and Thoroughbreds; one syndrome, multiple etiologies. Equine Vet J Suppl 30: 533-538.

Valentine, B.A. and B.J. Cooper, 2005. Incidence of polysaccharide storage myopathy: necropsy study of 225 horses. Vet Pathol 42: 823-827.

Monitoring orthopaedic health in competition horses

Sue Dyson[1] and Philippe Benoit[2]
[1]Centre for Equine Studies, Animal Health Trust, Lanwades Park, Kentford CB8 7UU Newmarket, Suffolk, United Kingdom; sue.dyson@aht.org.uk
[2]Philippe Benoit, Clinique Equine des Bréviaires, 78610 Les Breviaires, France; phbenoitdvm@aol.com

To write on monitoring the orthopaedic health in competition horses would be a book in itself. Thus, we had to decide to provide an exhaustive summary of the subject.

The aims of monitoring orthopaedic health are:

- prevention of orthopaedic injury
- early detection of problems and successful management
- recognition of a serious problem in a previously sound horse, that means the horse must be rested and cannot continue in work
- management of pre-existing problems
- recognition of a major problem in a horse near the end of it's career; can the problem be managed without a serious risk to welfare, to enable the horse to compete at a very important competition?

Prevention of orthopaedic injury

- horse selection
  - natural athletic ability – excessive athleticism may enhance risk
  - quality of paces
  - conformation
  - temperament and trainability
  - pain threshold
- knowledge of conformation and its influence on injury
  - foot
  - hock angle
  - hind fetlocks
  - length of back
- training programme and competition schedule
- work surfaces
- trimming and shoeing
- influence of the rider
- influence of the owner
  - monetary gain (short term)
  - compete at all costs

- gain necessary qualifications
- desire to save the horse for a special competition
- influence of the trainer
  - recognition of lameness
  - assumption that problem is training related
- prophylactic medication? e.g., oral nutraceuticals; intra-articular medication
- saddle fit
- monitoring also by physiotherapist
- experience of the veterinarian in dealing with orthopaedic injuries and the implications of injuries in different sport disciplines

Early detection of problems and successful management

- Knowing the rider and their abilities to detect, mask and/ or ignore problems
  - A strong and/ or very skilled rider may intuitively make corrections and be unaware of the problem e.g., minor lack of hindlimb engagement reflecting a pain related problem
  - A rider may attribute the problem to training
  - A rider may fail to recognise the significance of a problem e.g., landing with the right forelimb leading, although turning to the left
  - A rider may elect to ignore a problem
  - A rider may not intuitively think that minor reductions in performance may be pain related e.g., having rails down in front may reflect antebrachiocarpal joint pain
- Knowing the trainer and their abilities to detect, mask and/ or ignore problems
- Communication between trainer, rider and other professionals with the goal of optimising performance by managing minor problems
- Knowing the horse
  - Synovial effusion
  - Pain on passive flexion of a joint
  - Restriction of flexion of a joint
  - Positive response to flexion
  - Positive response to hoof testers
  - Muscle tension and/ or sensitivity
  - Flexibility of the neck and back
  - Reaction to pressure over the tubera sacrale
  - Reactivity to palpation of acupuncture points
  - Sensitivity to palpation of SDFT, DDFT, ALDDFT and SL
  - Flexibility of the neck
  - Stride length and elasticity
  - Balance and rhythm on the lunge on hard and soft surfaces

  - Behaviour when tacked up and mounted
  - Quality of paces under saddle
  - Quality of contact with the bit
  - Ease of flying changes and lateral work
  - Ability to collect and extend
  - Ease of turning to left and right
  - Natural jumping style
- Regular monitoring of the horse at home and sometimes in competition
- Good record keeping: comprehensive and accurate; the value of a work sheet for ease of documentation
- The potential value of intermittent video recording of gait
- Knowing the groom and their powers of observation; their ability to face reality and not 'bury their heads in the sand'; wanting the horse to be right; as opposed to wanting the horse to compete at all costs
  - Potential conflict of interest between loyalty to the rider and horse welfare

Recognition of a serious problem in a previously sound horse, that means the horse must be rested and cannot continue in work

- Certainty of diagnosis; the value of a second opinion
- Definitive localisation of pain and high quality imaging; no second guessing
- Knowledge of what constitutes a serious injury
- Knowledge of best treatment(s) and likely long term outcome

Management of pre-existing problems

- Accurate diagnosis
- Previous images
- Monitoring of lesion by serial clinical examinations and, if appropriate, diagnostic imaging e.g., radiography, ultrasonography, MRI
- When to examine the horse?
- Judicious medication
  - Which medication?
  - Timing of medication
  - Lack of knowledge of withdrawal times; 'moving the goal posts' by changing analytical methods
- Physical therapy
- Trimming and shoeing
- Warm up
- Work and competition schedule
- Work surfaces
- Working as a team with other professionals

- Knowledge of the athletic demands of the sport and which injuries can be managed for which sport
  - Dressage
  - Showjumping
  - Eventing
  - Endurance
  - Western performance

Recognition of a major problem in a horse near the end of it's career; can the problem be managed without a serious risk to welfare, to enable the horse to compete at a very important competition?

- Accurate diagnosis
- Knowledge of risks to the horse by continuation in work: the potential for catastrophic injury versus transient exacerbation of the problem

The problems of assessment of a horse of which you have no or limited prior knowledge

- Importance of communication with other professionals who have had prior dealings with horse: the veterinarian, the farrier, the physiotherapist.
- Access to previous clinical records and images.
- Not knowing what the horse has been living with.
- The advantages of a fresh set of eyes and hands and an unbiased appraisal.
- Getting the horse to the competition is not always in the best interests of the horse.
- The potential conflicts of interest between owners, riders, team managers and other clients.

The knowledge that there is always another professional person only too ready to disagree and to provide a short term fix.

The knowledge of the financial implications to the owner(s), rider, trainer and national federation.

The importance of professional ethics.

The importance of equine welfare.

The horse's foot as a source of poor performance

Tracy A. Turner
Anoka Equine Veterinary Services, Elk River, Minnesota, USA; turner@anokaequine.com

Foot and hoof lameness accounts for at least one-third of all chronic lamenesses in the horse. It must be understood that a digital nerve blocks simply localizes the source of the pain the horse senses to the foot. These horses' lameness will typically be improved by a palmar digital nerve block. It is important to identify as specifically as one can the pathological and clinical findings. This in turn will help the clinician make their best assessment of the problem, and recommend the most specific treatment.

There are numerous causes of pain in the foot of the horse. These causes can be arbitrarily divided into conditions of the hoof wall and horn producing tissues, conditions of the third phalanx, and conditions of the podotrochlear region. Hoof problems would include hoof wall defects, such as cracks or clefts that involve the sensitive tissue; any laminar tearing, separation or inflammation; contusions of the hoof causing bruising or corn formation; abscess formation; and pododermatitis (thrush or canker). Third phalanx lamenesses blocked out by a palmar digital anesthesia would include wing fractures, marginal fractures, solar fractures, or deep digital flexor insertional tenopathy. Conditions of the podotrochlear region have been reported to include distal interphalangeal synovitis, deep digital flexor tendinitis, desmitis of the impar (distal navicular ligament) or collateral sesamoidean ligaments, navicular osteitis or osteopathy, and vascular disease. The common denominator of all these conditions is that they are characterized by pain that can be localized to the caudal aspect of the hoof.

The first step in developing a logical approach to the treatment of palmar hoof pain is accurate assessment of the pain and careful evaluation of hoof structure that may predispose to or cause the pain. It is this author's opinion that a minimum of four diagnostic tests should be performed: hoof tester examination, distal limb flexion, hoof extension wedge test, and palmar hoof wedge test. A positive response to any of these tests is important but a negative response is equivocal and does not rule out any problem. Hoof tester examination should begin with systematic evaluation of the sole and then to the distal sesamoid region which includes the collateral sulci to opposite hoof wall, central sulcus to toe, and across the heels. A positive response should be repeatable, and in the distal sesamoid region the pain response should be uniform over those areas and must be evaluated in relation to examination of the remaining foot. That is, a positive response in the heels and quarters of the sole would also be expected to cause a positive response across the distal sesamoid region in the same area of the foot. Percussion utilizing a small hammer can also provide important information regarding pain in the hoof wall or sole.

Distal limb flexion test may exacerbate lameness if any of the three distal joints of the leg are affected by synovitis or osteoarthritis. A positive response could also be expected by any condition that causes induration of the tissues of the foot. This has been shown to be positive in over 95% of horses with navicular disease.

The hoof extension test is performed by elevating the toe with a block, holding the opposite limb, and trotting the horse away after 60 seconds. The palmar hoof wedge test is performed by placing the block under the palmar two-thirds of the frog and forcing the horse to stand on that foot. The test can be further modified so that the wedge can be placed under either heel to determine if the pressure there causes exacerbation of the lameness.

Typically, all these before mentioned lamenesses will be improved by at least 90% after perineural anesthesia of the palmar digital nerves but it does not help differentiate these lamenesses. Anesthesia of the distal interphalangeal (DIP) joint or the podotrochlear bursa are additional procedures that provide information about palmar hoof pain. In a study reported by Dyson, in 95% of the horses examined using DIP and bursa anesthesia, significant new information about the pain the horse exhibited was realized. The pain relief by anesthesia of any of these three regions has been shown to overlap. The DIP joint and podotrochlear bursa do not communicate, and yet the results of injecting anesthetic into these synovial cavities are similar. Both cavities have in common the navicular bone, the impar ligament, and the collateral sesamoidean ligament (proximal suspensory ligament of the navicular bone). The neuroreceptors for the navicular bone are in those 2 ligaments and they can be anesthetized from either synovial cavity. Further, Bowker showed that the palmar digital nerve is in very close proximity to the medial and lateral limits of the bursa and the nerve may be anesthetized at this level whenever the bursa is injected. Palmar foot pain can be divided into 5 groups, those horses with navicular region pain (desensitized by DIP analgesia and bursa analgesia, as well as palmar digital analgesia), those with distal interphalangeal pain (desensitized by DIP analgesia, as well as palmar digital analgesia but not bursa analgesia), those that are not desensitized by DIP analgesia but are desensitisized by bursa analgesia, as well as palmar digital analgesia, those that are improved by either DIP or bursa analgesia but are not sound but are sound after palmar digital analgesia, and those that are not desensitized by either DIP or bursal analgesia but are desensitized by palmar digital analgesia. It has also been noted recently that injection of the podotrochlear bursa can be very difficult and that it is quite easy to inject the DIP joint instead. We have found that not only is radiographic control necessary to successfully perform this block but that adding contrast media to the anesthetic to prove the limits of the block is also necessary.

This has lead to a new method of assessing navicular pathology, by evaluating the cartilage of the flexor surface of the navicular bone by contrast arthrography. Injection into the bursa was made from the palmar surface with the limb flexed at the carpus. Aseptic injection techniques were used to inject a 3 ml mixture of 1:1 contrast material and local anesthetic. The landmarks for needle insertion were just proximal to the central sulcus of the frog with the needle directed in line with the apex of the frog and in a direction parallel to the ground surface of the hoof. A 20 gauge 3.5 inch needle was used. The needle was inserted until resistance was encountered; this was usually at 2/3 the length of the needle. If the needle was inserted further it usually indicated incorrect placement. A lateral radiograph of the hoof was taken to confirm the position of the needle prior to injection. Ideally the needle should be midway between the proximal and distal borders. Once needle position was confirmed the bursa was injected with the contrast mixture and a second lateral hoof radiograph was taken to confirm filling of the bursa. If the bursa has been injected, then a PP-PD oblique projection of the navicular bone was obtained.

A distinct line of contrast material juxtaposed to the deep digital flexor tendon was normally separated from the navicular cortical bone by a layer of radiolucent fibrocartilage. Five basic findings were noted on contrast navicular bursography:

1. Normal flexor fibrocartilage.
2. Thinning or erosions of the flexor fibrocartilage (confirmed by post mortem examination in 3 cases).
3. Complete focal loss of the dye column which was thought to be due to flexor tendon adhesions to the bone (confirmed by post mortem in 2 cases).
4. Presence of flexor subchondral bone cystic defects which was noted as focal filling of the flexor cortical area with contrast.
5. Fibrillation of the deep flexor tendon which was noted as filling defects along the bursal surface of the deep flexor tendon. Normal fibrocartilage was seen in 13% of the examinations. Thinning or erosions of the flexor fibrocartilage was seen in 69% of the bursograms. Adhesions (loss of the dye column) were noted in 8% of the cases. Filling defects of the navicular flexor surface was noted in only 2% of the horses. Fibrillation of the deep flexor tendon was recognized in 21% of the horses. When the cases were divided between horses with navicular pain and palmar foot pain according to the criteria described by Turner more interesting comparisons could be made. Horses with normal flexor cartilage were more likely to have navicular pain (np) (8 of 97) rather than palmar foot pain (pfp) (5 of 97). This is in contrast to horses with cartilage thinning or erosions where horses with palmar foot

pain were more likely to exhibit this change (38/ 97 for pfp versus 29/97 for np). Horses thought to have adhesions, all were in the navicular pain group while there was no difference in horses with flexor filling defects (1/97pfp and 1/97np). Horses showing tendon fibrillation were also more likely to show palmar foot pain (14/97) rather than navicular pain (6/97). Contrast navicular bursography indicated pathology in the flexor cortex region 60% more often than plain film radiography.

Navicular bursography was devised due to the necessity to confirm injection of local anesthetic into the bursa. The bursa is not only a small space but is also in close proximity to other synovial structures such as the distal interphalangeal joint or distal tendon sheath. Because of this the bursa can be difficult to inject. Use of this technique allows one to know bursa injection has occurred. The contrast study was begun once it was realized that one could identify the flexor fibrocartilage of the navicular bone. After, the changes that were noted were simply identified and recorded for every case.

Interestingly, normal flexor fibrocartilage was noted more frequently in horses thought to have navicular pain. This finding tends to refute the long believed premise that navicular disease begins as damage to the flexor fibrocartilage or at the very least suggests that there may be more than one pathogenesis of navicular pain. Following these cases with subsequent bursography would be a method to follow the pathogenesis of these cases. To date, we have not repeated the bursography on any case.

The most common change noted on the bursograms was that of flexor cartilage thinning. However, when horses lame due to navicular pain were compared to horses lame due to other pain in the palmar foot there was no statistical difference between the 2 groups although the change occurs more frequently in the pfp group. This may reflect that this change is a normal wearing process or it may be either a primary or secondary response. Rooney has shown that toe first landing can lead to this change. Toe first landing may be seen with any cause of palmar foot pain. It would follow then that the change in biomechanics from the toe first landing is causing this change rather than some other biomechanical reason. The results of this study would tend to support that reasoning since this change was more common in pfp cases. Further, this would underline the importance of pain management in these cases in order to get the horse to load the foot correctly.

Adhesion formation was only noted in horses with navicular pain; whereas, flexor filling defects occurred equally in navicular as well as other causes of palmar foot pain. This indicates that the adhesions are associated with navicular pain but that defects on the flexor surface may be developmental and have no effect on pain. Lesions of the flexor surface of the deep flexor tendon have been noted and some have suggested that this may be an early navicular pathology. However, in this study fraying of the tendon was seen more than two times more often in the palmar foot pain group. In most cases, tendon fraying was associated with flexor fibrocartilage thinning and erosions (12 of 20 cases). At this time no speculation can be made which came first.

Overall, navicular bursography is a simple technique that can be used to confirm injection into the navicular bursa and can also give valuable new information regarding pathology in the region of the navicular bone. A change seen via contrast navicular bursography represent stages of pathologic damage and allows more timely therapeutic intervention and more accurate prognostication. The author's approach to these types of cases is to develop a treatment strategy based on the individual case needs rather than a treatment formula. Bursography has improved the ability to identify pathology such as flexor cartilage erosions and to utilize therapy such as chondroprotective agents, identification of tendon injuries causes concern for tendinitis and strict rest to allow healing of the tendon can be instituted and the identification of adhesions has been a grave prognostic indicator for conservative management. This technique also provides a means to study the pathogenesis of navicular disease or navicular pathology because it provides important information about anatomical structures that have only been able to be evaluated at post mortem. By utilizing this technique we can further our understanding of navicular problems.

Recently it has become possible to examine the podotrochlear region sonographically. In order to examine the podotrochlea the superficial horn must be prepared from the frog to expose soft, spongy frog tissue. Next, sonographic gel is liberally applied to the frog. The ultrasound transducer is then applied to the frog. Images of the podotrochlea are apparent from the center of the frog to the apex. A 7.5 MHZ probe provides the best image.

Generally, at the center third of the frog, the flexor surface of the navicular bone is readily noticeable as a hyper echoic line. The bursa is seen as a hypo echoic (fluid filled) region juxtaposed to the navicular bone. The deep flexor fibers can be seen curving around the bone. As the probe is moved toward the apex of the frog, the distal aspect of the navicular bone can be identified as can the intersection between the deep flexor tendon and the impar ligament. As the probe reaches the apex of the frog the deep flexor's insertion on the third phalanx becomes apparent.

Ultrasound is an excellent means to visualize soft tissue structures. However, examination of the foot has been limited to the pastern because the hoof capsule served as a barrier to examination of the hoof. The proximal regions of the navicular bone could be examined if one had a special probe that would fit between the bulbs of the horse's heels. However, this gave no information as to what may be occurring further distally. The frog however, because of its high water content can serve as the hoof's 'stand off'. By removing the hard, outer layers this exposes tissue that can transmit sound waves allowing the examiner to see this distal tissues.

Radiography of the navicular bone includes a minimum of 5 projections of each foot, the D65Pr-PaDiO, the D45Pr-PaDiO, the lateral to medial, the PaPr-PaDiO projection, and a horizontal DP projection. Projections are assessed for changes of the navicular bone including enlarged synovial fossa, enthesiopathy, cyst-like formations, or changes of the flexor cortical region. Radiographic examination is the imaging method most often used to assess osseous changes in the distal sesamoid bone and third phalanx. These changes with the exception of fractures are usually not pathognomonic but do provide insight into damage that has occurred to the foot. Fractures also may not be radiographically visible until 10 to 14 days after the injury occurred.

Scintigraphy is a technique that measures gamma ray emission from a radioactive nuclide injected into the animal. The technique provides information on relative vascularity and rate of tissue metabolism. This is particularly useful in studying bone pathology and can help differentiate sites of injury in the foot.

Thermography provides information regarding skin temperature. It has been shown to be useful in assessing the relative blood flow to a region. This information is of particular interest when pre- and post-exercise temperatures are determined. Exercise will normally cause a 0.5 °C rise in skin temperature. Whenever, the skin temperature does not rise, poor blood flow should be considered a factor in the disease being assessed.

As part of the overall evaluation of these horses an objective assessment of hoof balance is important. Eleven measurements are made of each foot. The horse's weight is determined with a weight tape or scale. Seven measurements are made of the hoof length with a tape measure: medial and lateral heel lengths, medial and lateral quarter lengths, dorsomedial and dorsolateral toe lengths, and sagittal toe length. These measurements are recorded on a graph to illustrate the general shape of the foot. In addition, the frog's length and width are measured at their longest and widest points. The hoof circumference immediately below the coronary band, and the hoof angle (using a hoof gauge) are also measured. From these measurements, two additional measurements can be calculated: the frog ratio (frog width divided by length) and the body size to hoof area (horse's weight (pounds) X 12.56 / square of the hoof wall circumference(C) (inches)).

After plotting the hoof wall lengths, one should have a curve that reflects the shape of the hoof. For a hoof of average hoof angle (48°-55°), flattening of the plotted curve indicates that the heels are underrun. A flat curve would also be expected for very upright hooves (>60°). Generally speaking, the 3 measurements at the toe should be equal. The measurements at the quarter are usually 1-2 cm shorter than the toe (for the average hoof). The heel length should generally be about one-third of the toe length. The remaining measurements are used in the previously described formulas to determine weight to body size and frog ratios for determination of a contracted foot.

A dorsopalmar (plantar) and a lateral radiograph of the hoof can also be used to determine valuable information about hoof balance. The horse must be standing with the metacarpus (tarsus) perpendicular to the ground which can most easily be determined by either the use of a level placed against the cannon bone or the use of a weighted string to align the leg. The radiographic beam should be horizontal and centered on the hoof. Resting the horse's foot on a block to raise the hoof off the ground facilitates these exposures (the opposite limb should be similarly elevated). For easy identification of landmarks, radiopaque markers can be attached to the hoof. A wire placed sagittally (midline) along the toe from the coronary band to the ground, a thumb tack in the apex of the frog and thumb tacks in the most caudal point of the ground contact of each heel emphasize these areas on the radiographs, making their identification much easier.

Lateral to medial (LM) and dorsopalmar (DP) views of the horse's feet are needed to assess hoof balance. The radiographs were used to determine measurements of dorsopalmar hoof balance (LM projections) and medial to lateral hoof balance (DP projections). LM projections are evaluated for:

1. Hoof angle by measuring the angle produced by the intersection of the dorsal hoof wall with the ground.
2. Heel angle determined by a line from the caudal aspect of the hairline to the heel ground contact.
3. Palmar angle of the coffin bone is measured by a line drawn from the toe of the bone to the wings along the palmar border, the angle is determined by the intersection of this line with a line parallel to the ground surface.
4. Coffin bone angle is determined by a line parallel to the dorsal surface of the third phalange and its intersection with a line parallel to the ground.
5. Toe-heel support ratio is determined by dropping a perpendicular line down from the coffin-joint's center of articulation (COA) and expressing toe measurement over heel measurement.
6. Phalangeal bone alignment is determined by the rotational position of the coffin and pastern joints which are the centers of these bones. Lines are drawn through the centers of the first and second phalanges. A line parallel to the dorsal surface of the third phalange determines the line of the coffin bone.

7. DP projections are used to assess medial to lateral balance.
8. The hoof is equal side to side from the midline by measuring the distance from the middle of the central sulcus to the widest point of the medial hoof capsule and comparing to the distance from central sulcus to the lateral wall at the widest distance.
9. Joint alignment is assessed using the DP radiograph and drawing lines through the medial and lateral aspects of the three distal joints. If the lines are parallel the angle between the lines is zero
10. Coffin bone levelness is assessed by drawing a line along the distal aspect of the coffin bone between medial and lateral wings. If the angle this line makes with the ground is zero the coffin bone is level.

Additional hoof balance information is possible with simple calculations.
1. Underrun heel calculation is made by subtracting heel angle from hoof angle. Ideally the number should be zero, cut off has been made at 5°.1
2. Hoof capsule deviation is determined by subtracting the coffin bone angle from the hoof angle. Ideally this should be zero.
3. The toe-heel support ratio is computed by dividing the distance from the COA point to the toe as a percent of the length from toe to heel at the ground level. Ideally this should be 50%.
4. Medial lateral balance is equal side to side from the midline can be calculated by determining a percentage ratio off a DP radiograph, the distance from the middle of the central sulcus to the widest point of the medial hoof capsule compared to the distance from medial to lateral wall at the widest distance, medial width is measured as a percentage of the whole width. If lateral to medial balance is equal the percentage will be 50%.

Examination of the lateral and dorsopalmar (plantar)(DP) radiographs provides excellent pictorial evidence of imbalance. The lateral radiograph should be evaluated for P2 and P3 alignment which gives insight into the presence of a broken-hoof axis. In addition, the alignment between P3 and the hoof wall should be assessed. If the hoof wall and dorsal surface of P3 are not parallel the functional hoof angle can be determined by measuring the angle of the dorsal surface of P3 with the ground. Usually the slope of the heels can be seen on the radiograph and can also be used to determine whether the heels are underrun.

The DP radiographic projection should be assessed for joint alignment, medial and lateral hoof wall lengths, and foot symmetry. Joint alignment is determined by examining the symmetry of the joint space. Malalignment is present if one side of the joint is more narrow. This phenomenon can also be caused by poor positioning in which case all three of the lower leg joints (fetlock, pastern, and coffin) will be affected. The hoof wall length can be measured directly from the film. The symmetry of weight bearing can be predicted in a similar manner.

LM projection concepts

1. Hoof angle ranged between 51° and 56°.
2. Heel angle ranged from 30° to 67°.
3. The palmar coffin bone angle ranged between 1.5° to 6°.
4. Coffin bone angle should be between 50° to 54°.
5. Toe-heel support ratio for our normals was 62-70%.
6. The coffin joint axis had a mean of 8.27° extension and the pastern had a mean of 5.78° extension.

DP projection concepts

7. Hoof symmetry was very close with a mean of 49% medial 51% lateral.
8. The coffin and pastern joints are parallel in mature non lame horses.
9. The distal aspect of the coffin bone should be parallel to the ground. There was a tendency for horses at the end of their shoeing/trimming cycle to be slightly higher (longer) on the lateral side.

Calculated measures

Determining underrun heels showed that the mean difference was 8.3°. This is much greater than the ideal zero and higher than previously reported for upper limit of normal. Hoof capsule deviation showed that normally the number should be zero but horses with coffin bone rotation had a negative number and horses where the dorsal hoof wall thickness was wider proximally than distally had a positive number. Toe-heel ratio by tradition should have been 50% but it was not. Most horses were between 62-70% toe over heel. Finally the symmetric hoof measure was 49%, very close to the traditional 50%.

Through thorough examination of the horse affected by pain in the palmar region of the foot a more precise diagnosis can be made, whether the diagnosis reflects injury to the hoof capsule, third phalanx, or podotrochlear region. Treatment then should be based on the type of injury. Thorough examination of the horse affected with navicular syndrome is important not only to determine that the horse has the syndrome but also to try to determine which type of disease process is at work. Treatment then should be based on the type of injury.

Some useful references

Balch, O., K.K. White and D. Butler, 1991. Factors involved in the balancing of equine hooves. J Am Vet Med Assoc 198: 1980-1989.

Bowker, R., K. Linder and K. Van Wulfen, 1997. Anatomy of the distal interphalangeal joint of the mature horse: relationships with the navicular suspensory ligaments, sensory nerves and neurovascular bundle. Equine Vet J 29: 126-129.

Dyson, S. and L. Kidd, 1993. A comparison of responses to analgesia of the navicular bursa and intra-articular analgesia of the distal interphalangeal joint in 59 horses. Equine Vet J 25: 93.

Dyson, S., 2002. Subjective and quantitative scintigraphic assessment of the equine foot and its relationship with hoof pain. Equine Vet J 34: 164-169.

Dyson, S. and D. Marks, 2003. Foot pain and the elusive diagnosis. in O'Grady SE (ed): Podiatry, Vet Clin of NA: Eq Prac, Philadelphia, WB Saunders Co, 19: 531-565.

Pool, R.R., D.M. Meagher and S.M. Stover, 1989. Pathophysiology of navicular syndrome. Vet Clin No Am, Eq Pract 5: 109-129.

Poulos, P.W., and M.F. Smith, 1988. The nature of enlarged vascular channels in the navicular bone of the horse. Vet Radiol 29: 60-64.

Rijkenhuizen, A., F. Nemeth, K.J. Dik and S.A. Goedegebuure, 1989. The arterial supply of the navicular bone in adult horses with navicular disease. Equine Vet J 21: 418.

Sage, A.M. and T.A. Turner, 2000. Ultrasonography in the horse with palmar foot pain: 13 cases. In Proceedings Am Assoc Equine Practnr, 46: 380-381.

Sage, A.M. and T.A. Turner, 2002. Ultrasonography of the soft tissue of the equine foot. Equine Vet Educ 4: 278-283.

Turner, T.A., S.K. Kneller and R.R. Badertscher, 1986. Radiographic changes in the navicular bone of normal horses. in Proceedings Am Assoc Equine Practnr 32: 309-316.

Turner, T.A. and C. Stork, 1988. Hoof abnormalities and their relation to lameness. In Proceedings Am Assoc Equine Practnr, 34: 293-297.

Turner, T.A., 1989. Diagnosis and treatment of the navicular syndrome in horses. In: J.V. Yovich (Ed) The Equine Foot, Vet Clin of NA: Eq Prac, Philadelphia, WB Saunders Co, p. 131-144.

Turner, T.A., 1992. The use of hoof measurements for the objective assessment of hoof balance. In Proceedings Am Assoc of Equine Practnr, 38: 157-164.

Turner, T.A., 1996.: Predictive value of diagnostic tests for navicular pain. In Proceedings Am Assoc Equine Practnr 42: 201.

Turner, T.A., 1996. Differentiation of navicular region pain from other forms of palmar heel pain. Pferdeheilkunde, 12: 603-606.

Turner, T.A., 1998. Use of navicular bursography in 97 horses. In Proceedings Am Assoc Equine Practnr 44: 227-230.

Turner, T.A., 2002. Desmitis of the distal interphalangeal collateral ligaments: 22 cases.. In Proceedings Am Assoc Equine Practnr, 48: 343-346.

Turner, T.A., 2003. Examination of the equine foot. In: S.E. O'Grady (Ed): Podiatry, Vet Clin of NA: Eq Prac, Philadelphia, WB Saunders Co, 19: 309-332.

Wright, I., 1993. A study of 118 cases of navicular disease: clinical features. Equine Vet J 25: 488.

Wright, I., 1993. A study of 118 cases of navicular disease: radiological features. Equine Vet J 25: 493.

Could it be the foot? If yes, what can be done?

Andrew P. Bathe
Rossdales Equine Hospital, Cotton End Road, Exning, Newmarket, Suffolk, CB8 7NN, United Kingdom; andy.bathe@rossdales.com

Introduction

This article will try to cover the scenario of the poorly performing Sport Horse within two weeks of an important competition. My experience is based upon treating event, dressage and show jumping horses, extending from recreational to elite level. Horses and ponies will often have specific targets within a season, whether it be Pony Club camp or the Olympics. The scenario of an acute onset of a performance-limiting problem prior to a major competition is most common in event horses because their work level will usually peak twice a year for major three-day-events, whereas for dressage and show jumping the level of work tends to be somewhat more constant. Poor performance may be due to the acute onset of a new problem, or may be due to the continuation or exacerbation of an underlying, low-grade problem. The distinction between these can be blurred as many injuries in Sports Horses are repetitive strain injuries and even acute presentation may have had an insidious onset with prodromal signs being present, even if only in retrospect. Thus my major strategy when dealing with maintenance of advanced level horses at the top level is to avoid this scenario as much as possible. This paper will concentrate on the acute presentation of a fresh injury.

Lameness is, in my experience, the most common cause of poor performance in Sport Horses. It is more common for hindlimb lameness to be presented as poor performance because riders find it more difficult to identify the presence of lameness and the horse may simply present with a lack of impulsion or power. Forelimb lameness is more easily identified and will often present as such rather than as a loss of performance. However, good riders subconsciously adjust for any irregularities in the horse's gait and can be quite successful at masking low-grade forelimb lameness.

Could it be the foot?

The foot is a common site of acute-onset pain and should always be considered as a lameness differential. The level of diagnostic investigation will vary depending upon how obvious the clinical signs are, but with presentation immediately prior to a major competition the investigations may be less extensive than when there is no time pressure. The history for an event horse presenting with foot lameness would normally be either lameness itself or stopping at drop fences, especially on hard ground. There may be a history of external trauma, such as hitting a fence or of having lost a shoe. The onset of the problem relative to the last shoeing should be noted. Three Day Event horses are normally shod approximately seven days before a major competition so the clenches will still be tight, but there is time to deal with any lameness arising as a consequence of shoeing. Show jumpers with foot lameness may present with a reluctance to jump or sometimes, more specifically, a reluctance to land on a certain lead over a fence. There is rarely a feeling of lack of power, which is more common presentation for hindlimb lameness. In dressage horses there may be a reluctance to fully extend or to work on a particular rein.

In terms of clinical examination, evaluation of digital pulse amplitude is a more reliable indicator of foot inflammation than manually assessing the hoof temperature. The foot confirmation, horn quality and style of shoeing should be carefully assessed. Thorough use of hoof testers is mandatory, even in cases where the foot is not suspected as a cause of the problem. Diagnostic local analgesia may be necessary to confirm the foot as the source of pain and I would normally allow a five day withdrawal period for local anaesthetics prior to competition and do try to avoid using large volumes. The emphasis is generally upon being minimally invasive close to competition and perineural analgesia carries a low risk of complications. A palmar digital nerve block will be positive in many horses with foot pain, but it should be noted that many cases of pain located in the digit do not fully block out until an abaxial sesamoid nerve block is performed. Distal interphalangeal joint analgesia is relatively straightforward and can guide therapeutic options, and indeed blocking may be combined with speculative treatment with corticosteroids. A navicular bursal block is relatively invasive in comparison and I would be reluctant to perform this immediately prior to competition when there will be pressure to not clip the horse, which can compromise the asepsis of the technique. The proximal interphalangeal joint should not be forgotten, especially in horses that block better to abaxial sesamoid than a palmar digital nerve block.

Thermography can be an extremely useful, non-invasive way of accurately determining blood flow and superficial inflammation within the foot. Radiography will be employed in a standard fashion. With an acute presentation of lameness, wing fractures of the pedal bone or gas shadows from a subsolar abscess may be detected. In more insidious onset lameness, good quality palmaroproximal- and palmarodistal oblique (flexor view) projections are mandatory. Ultrasonographic examination has a role in assessing the collateral ligaments of the distal interphalangeal joint and the palmar soft tissue structures in the pastern region. It is also possible to identify the digital flexor tendon and the navicular bone through the frog, but in all these methods of assessment there is incomplete visualisation of the soft tissue structures. It can be useful if there is a clearly identified lesion, but negative findings cannot rule out the presence of significant pathology. Thus I do not consider it a high yield technique unless there are signs of localised swelling to guide the evaluation and interpretation of any suspicious findings. Gamma scintigraphic examination can be very helpful in acute onset severe lameness arising from the foot, with no radiographic changes. This is relatively non-invasive, but the horse has to be taken out of exercise whist it is radioactive and hospitalised. The biggest recent advancement in the diagnosis of foot pathology is undoubtedly standing MRI examination, and this is highly applicable in this scenario. The horse does require heavy sedation, but again, the withdrawal period for these products does not really extend beyond 5-7 days. The level of anatomic detail and information about the type of pathology and activity present is far superior to any other imaging modality. It is possible to rule in or out the presence of a significant soft tissue injury within the foot, such as collateral ligament or DDFT injuries. Acute bone oedema in the phalanges or navicular bone can also be identified.

Conditions

The most common conditions presenting with this scenario are superficial foot pain from corns and subsolar abscesses. Problems seem most common in Three Day Event horses in the spring, and often do present two weeks before Badminton Horse Trials. The change in weather from wet to dry(er) at this time of year can be a predisposing factor. Palmar foot pain, predisposed by poor foot conformation and shoeing can also become more apparent as the plane of exercise peaks. Any of the standard causes of more chronic foot pain can also present acutely. The important differentiation is between coffin joint or navicular pain, which may be responsive to treatment and the horse may be able to continue to exercise without risk of significant exacerbation of the injury, versus an acute soft tissue injury, in which case it would be contraindicated to allow the horse to continue exercise. As stated earlier, MRI enables us to answer these questions quite accurately. The clinical presentation can also give significant clues, as coffin joint or navicular pain will often be more obvious on a hard surface, whereas soft tissue injuries can be evident on a soft surface, even in the leg on the outside and will often lead riders to think that there is more upper limb injury.

Treatment

Foot related lameness does offer a number of therapeutic options. Acute inflammation will be often treated to try and minimise the degree of inflammation. In cases of solar abscesses the aim should be to try and encourage maturation of the infection and encourage drawing of the infection to the surface. Thus poulticing and hot tubing can be very useful and if an abscess is developing it is often better in the long term to be patient and allow it to come to surface rather than making large defects into the wall or sole at an early stage. I will often prepare a small area for drainage and it can be possible to lavage thoroughly in a minimally invasive fashion. The degree of inflammation associated with superficial foot infections can be considerable and I would administer high levels of anti-inflammatory drugs, whilst taking care to observe the withdrawal times and proximity of competition. Once the acute inflammation has subsided, the shoe will be replaced and the horse should not be put back into full work for another few days to again allow the inflammation to fully subside. The defect must be kept clean and dry. Unloading areas of sensitivity, such as by floating in the heel, use of a bar shoe or solar packing material can be extremely helpful, but this is not the time to instigate massive changes in the horse's way of shoeing and the response to any change must be carefully assessed. The use of studs should be minimised during this period.

Treatment of acute soft tissue injuries to try and mask them through the competition is not appropriate. However, medication of the coffin joint can be effective if there is a good block response in this area. I use a withdrawal period of approximately two weeks for triamcinolone and the long withdrawal period for methylprednisolone acetate means it is not a sensible choice within these time periods. FEI testing for betamethasone is extremely sensitive and thus it is not a good drug of choice. The withdrawal period for dexamethasone is short, at around three-four days and this can have applicability in treatment close to competition. I usually combine this with hyaluronic acid (HA) and I do not find that HA on its own offers any great benefit. A recent product which gets around the issues of withdrawal periods is autologous conditioned serum (IRAP). This product contains anti-inflammatory proteins and can have applicability in the treatment of horses with joint disease close to competition. Extra corporeal shockwave therapy can have some analgesic action, either used in treating the area of pain or by using it over the palmar digital nerves.

Prevention

As mentioned in the introduction, I would consider a horse presenting with poor performance prior to competition to often be a failure of good rider and veterinary management. The emphasis upon managing these horses is to try and prevent this very scenario from occurring. My elite-level horses would normally have a thorough veterinary examination at least twice a year and any low-grade problems are evaluated and treated without concerns of proximity to competition. A high quality of farriery must be maintained and this can be difficult for show jumpers and dressage horses as they are often travelling round Europe on a competitive circuit rather than having one consistent farrier. In horses with pain responsive to medication of the coffin joints, these would often be routinely treated three weeks or so prior to a major competition.

Conclusions

Poor performance and lameness can arise from the foot in the run up to an important competition. This can present a different set of challenges to the standard lameness evaluation and treatment, but with good teamwork between the vet, farrier and rider, it can be possible to enable the horse to achieve its intended target. The bonus is often upon us as veterinary surgeons to determine those situations in which it would be inappropriate to try and continue the horse in exercise. The emphasis in the management of elite horses should always be towards preventing this scenario happening however.

Further reading

Bathe, A.P., 2002. Chronic Foot Lameness. In: S. Curtis (Ed.) Corrective Farriery: a textbook of remedial horseshoeing Volume I Newmarket: R&W Publications Ltd. P. 81-104.

Bathe, A.P. and S. Curtis, 2006. Acute Foot Lameness In: S. Curtis (Ed.) Corrective Farriery: a textbook of remedial horseshoeing Volume II Newmarket: R&W Publications Ltd. p. 585-602.

Bathe, A.P., Lameness in the three day event horse In: M.W. Ross and S.J. Dyson (Eds.) Diagnosis and management of lameness in the horse Philadelphia: Saunders, p. 984-996.

Acquired neurological conditions of performance horses in the 'peri-event period'

Lutz Goehring[1] and Barrie Grant[2]
[1]Colorado State University, Fort Collins, Colorado, USA; Lutz.Goehring@ColoState.edu
[2]San Luis Rey Equine Hospital, Bonsall, California, USA; barriegrant@earthlink.net

The premise of challenge of this presentation is to discuss the more common conditions that can result in neurological deficits and clinical signs in horses that previously were performing well. We hope to discuss the typical history, clinical presentation, specific diagnostic tests, recommendations for treatment and prognosis. We will first attempt to separate the more common causes into two groups 1. Those caused by infectious or toxic agents and 2. Those caused by trauma or physical abnormalities to the head, spinal column or peripheral nerves.

Group 1 (summarized by Lutz Goehring)

We have to recognize that an increased risk for performance horses exists to contract neurological disease caused by either infection or intoxication during the period of going to, being at and returning from an event. When we compare performance horses with those that stay at home there is the risk of transportation, and the risk of a different, new environment upon arrival. 'Transportation' is a risk factor not only for mechanically induced trauma, but it induces in addition a less well-defined syndrome of 'transportation stress'. This syndrome decreases the efficacy of the immune system; it may impair mucociliary clearance in the respiratory tract, and may also alter a horse's gastro-intestinal flora because of changes in food and water intake. Besides a decreased efficacy of the innate or aspecific arm of the immune system the specific arm is neither prepared for specific pathogens nor toxins upon exposure. Immunologically naïve horses, horses with fading vaccination titers, or non-vaccinated horses will be an easy target for locally specific pathogens. Therefore, it is important that necessary **homework** is done long before horses go on transport to an event. This becomes in particular important the further away the horse travels.

Homework:

- What pathogens are relevant for the region or area that is visited?
- Are there safe and efficacious vaccines available, and what is the vaccination schedule?
- What are the odds: is there a relevant risk of exposure to pathogens or toxins?
- What alternative or additional measures can be taken to minimize the risk of exposure, uptake of a toxin or infection with a pathogen?

Infectious agents with subsequent neurological outcome

Typical features for an infection leading to neurological disease in horses are: (1) **asymmetrical** presentation of clinical neurological signs; (2) changes of the CSF composition; (3) several horses (more than 1) show clinical signs at the same time, possibly only a fever.

As an example let's take a look at the dressage horse from Belgium that is planning to go to a competition in Lexington, Kentucky, USA in February 2009. The following infectious diseases with neurological outcome are endemic to this region of the United States, and may be encountered: Equine Protozoal Myeloencephalitis (EPM) caused by the protozoan *Sarcocystis neurona*, Togavirus encephalitis (Eastern Equine Encephalitis virus, EEE), Flavivirus encephalitis/myelitis (West Nile virus, WNV), Rabies virus encephalitis/myelitis (Rabies virus). The only vaccination this horse may already have, and covering diseases in the US is a Rabies vaccination. In general, Rabies vaccines provide a good level of protection. The chance of an encounter with a rabid animal, raccoon or skunk, is extremely small, and horses competing at the level described here will not be turned out into pasture during the event, which further decreases the chance of exposure.

Both, EEE and WNV are vector (mosquito)-transmitted diseases, and technically the immunologically naïve horse from Europe would be susceptible to these diseases. However, the competition is scheduled during the winter season, and it is therefore unlikely that infected mosquitoes will form a threat to this horse (and its rider, because both viruses are zoonotic diseases!). Very efficient and safe vaccines are available against EEE and WNV; however, the necessity of vaccination under these particular and well-defined circumstances would be debatable.

EPM is contracted by ingestion of *Sarcocystis neurona* oocysts which accumulate in the environment through fecal droppings of an opossum, a species found only in America. These animals are garbage eaters, scavengers of food of various kinds. Opossums find dog or cat food very tasty, and they may also consume horse feed, pellets and concentrate. Oocysts from *S. neurona*, upon ingestion by the horse, may rarely infect the central nervous system. It is estimated that in about 10 – 15 out of 10,000 horses the protozoan enters the CNS after ingestion and sporulation of oocysts in the GI tract. However, immunologically naïve horses are more susceptible, and horses from Europe in general are immunologic naïve because *S. neurona* is restricted to the American continent. The risk of ingestion of oocysts, can be minimized by avoiding pasture access and increased diligence with feeding. Although there are protozoan-cidal drugs available (ponazuril, nitazoxanide, diclazuril) for the treatment of an acquired central nervous system infection with *S. neurona*, these drugs are not advised to be given as a preventative because of potential side effects and the relative small risk to become infected under the given circumstances.

Equine Herpesvirus type 1 (EHV-1) was not listed among the diseases described earlier, although EHV-1 is endemic to the United States. The reason is that probably all (performance) horses world-wide are latent carrier of EHV-1, and no adult horses should be considered 'immunologically naïve' for EHV-1. The Belgian dressage horse may in fact 'reencounter' EHV-1 during his trip to the US by 2 distinct pathways: the horse may recrudesce or re-activate EHV-1 from its latent state and location because of travel stress, which will be followed by viral replication in the upper respiratory tract. Alternatively, the horse may become horizontally infected by another horse which is already shedding virus into the environment through its respiratory tract. The disease that may follow and cause central nervous system damage is called Equine Herpesvirus-associated myeloencephalopathy or **EHM**. Viral replication in the respiratory epithelium is followed by a translocation of virus into nearby lymphnodes, where lymphocytes will become infected. Upon recirculation of lymphocytes virus is transported within cells in the blood stream: **cell-associated viremia**. What follows is not completely understood; however, interaction between infected lymphocytes and endothelial cells of the spinal cord leads to translocation of virus into the endothelial cell, which in some cases results in a vascular reaction, characterized by vasculitis and thrombosis. Perfusion failure of focal parts of the central nervous system will lead to ischemia and loss of function.

EHM is a typical winter and early spring disease, and is more likely to occur in tall breeds (Standardbred, Thoroughbred, Warmblood, Draught horse, Arabian, American Quarter Horse) rather than ponies. Cell-associated viremia is a prerequisite for EHM; however, only a fraction of viremic horses will develop EHM.

Spread of virus and infection of other horses is through droplet infection. Recent outbreak observations have shown that close nose-to-nose contact between horses is necessary for spread of infection, and fomites (hands, gear, clothes, etc) must play an intricate role in infection of others. Horses are febrile during viremia. Some may also show mild temperature increase during the initial respiratory tract infection. Fevers are therefore the first indicator of an infection possibly caused by EHV-1. *Because of the dramatic consequences of EHV-1 it cannot be emphasized enough how important it is to take a rectal temperature at least once daily in a horse preparing for a competition, twice daily in horses during a competition, followed by at least once daily temperature measurements when back home.* Regardless of the cause of a fever the horse should be promptly isolated. The cause of the fever should be determined, and 'taking temperatures' in neighboring horses should be intensified. Many diagnostic laboratories offer

PCR technology to determine the presence of (respiratory) pathogens in horses. These tests are reliable and have a fast turn-around time (days).

Although there are a variety of killed and modified-live vaccines against EHV-1 on the market they are only partially effective. None has a claim to prevent from neurological disease. These vaccines may decrease viral replication in the respiratory tract and therefore limit spread of disease, and, in addition, may decrease the quantitative aspect of viremia.

Toxins with neurological outcome:

Typical features of an intoxication causing neurological disease are: i) there is typically more than one horse affected; ii) a fever is extremely uncommon; iii) the presentation of neurological deficits is symmetrical.

Toxins can originate from 5 different sources: **feed, water, bedding**, and intentionally or unintentionally **applied substances**. A growing number of riders bring their own feed provided this is feasible. In other cases competition participants have to rely on the event organizers and their judgment and ability to provide quality feed material for the show. However, riders and grooms should be instructed and trained to check the quality of feed that is offered.

Although skin conditions such as blisters and ulceration of mucous membranes or urticarial reactions have been described in the literature upon contact with stall bedding material, reports on neurological disease induced by 'contaminated' bedding were not found. Water from public water supply should be safe. Water from a well or water from standing waters or ponds may form a risk. These waters may contain toxins such as botulism toxins or blue algae toxins, and the consumption should be avoided.

Feed material: in the past it became more popular to feed ensiled products to performance horses, in particular horses with a history of recurrent airway obstruction or inflammatory airway disease. Botulism is more often associated with silage feeding to horses. Ingestion of botulism toxin, which is commonly preformed in silage, has an extremely unfavorable outcome for horses. Toxins are absorbed from the GI tract and translocated to the storage vesicles located in the end plates of peripheral motor nerves. Botulism toxin inhibits the release of the neurotransmitter acetylcholine, and causes generalized weakness and paralysis in a horse. Cranial nerve function is impaired. A horse with clinical botulism will chew very slowly on its grain, and the tongue, when pulled out of its mouth and held tight for 30 sec, it will only gradually and with difficulties pull back the tongue into its mouth. Regurgitation may be noticed and potentially a nasal discharge mixed with feed particles is visible. Horses with botulism intoxication spend long hours in recumbency, and have difficulties to get up. Due to increasing muscle fatigue, horses with botulism show muscle fasciculations in the quadriceps and triceps area, and they suddenly collapse when muscle fatigue becomes overwhelming. Restoration of neuromuscular function requires the assembly of newly produced vesicles filled with neurotransmitter, and this may take up to 14 days. Survival is dose-dependent, and also depends on the demeanor of the horse whether or not the horse accepts long periods in lateral recumbency. Large doses will cause diaphragmatic paralysis, and the horse is unable to breathe. Although antitoxin is available, when administered it will only bind circulating toxin molecules, and not those bound already to the neurotransmitter vesicles. Immediate feed exchange and potentially treating horses that consumed silage from the same bale with anti-toxin should be the immediate action.

Against general opinion equine botulism is less frequently associated with a cadaver found in silage or hay, but it is more often associated with poor quality silage which did not go through an adequate acidification process. *Clostridium botulinum* spores, commonly found in soil, end up in the grass which will undergo the ensiling process and the bacteria will be able to sporulate under anaerobic conditions within the bale. It is therefore extremely critical to recognize silage as a vulnerable product, and silage should be inspected thoroughly prior to feeding in particular if it does not come from a known source. If silage is a regular part of a horse's diet it may be warranted to vaccinate the horse against *Clostridium botulinum* toxins. If one wants to provide a dust-free roughage diet to competition horses, however wants to avoid the risk of botulism, hay can also be thoroughly soaked and fed semi-moist to horses.

Hay can be another source of toxins which will affect the equine nervous system. Hay may contain tremorogens such as lolitrem (perennial ryegrass) or paspalitrems (Dallis grass, Bahia grass). Both groups of toxins interfere with the release of the inhibitory neurotransmitter GABA in the central nervous system, and cause significant hypermetria and muscle fasciculations. The hay which contains the toxins appears to be of good quality, and bales are relatively recently processed.

Clinical signs develop within a day after ingestion, and are dose-dependent. Horses are irritable; they tremble and are showing muscle fasciculations and hypermetria, and clinical signs may worsen with exercise. Exchanging the horse's feed will make signs disappear within a few days up to a week.

Environmental toxins causing neurological disease in horses are many; however, they are rarely reported, frequently because of a lack of causation. Examples of environmental toxins are methyl bromide used as a soil fumigant, carbamates, mercury, lead, strychnine (rodenticides), metaldehyde and methiocarb (molluscicides), 4-aminopyridine (bird repellant), amitraz (ectoparacidal), and organophosphates (insecticides).

Non-forage associated plant toxins are too numerous to list. Horses may become exposed to toxic weeds on a warm-up or cool-down ride around the event premises. Riders and grooms should be instructed to not allow a horse to feed on shrubs, bushes, plants along the way.

For all insults to the nervous system of a horse it is of utmost importance to get a detailed and candid history of recent events. Questions should be included that target the possible administration of 'forbidden substances', and in particular tranquilizing drugs (ask for fluphenazine!). 'History' becomes even more important when only a single horse is showing clinical signs. A thorough questioning should include the groom, the rider, the owner and, if during an event, contact should be established with the barn veterinarian at home.

For all insults to the nervous system of a horse it is of utmost importance to get a detailed and candid history of recent events. Questions should be included that target the possible administration of 'forbidden substances', and in particular tranquilizing drugs (ask for fluphenazine!). 'History' becomes even more important when only a single horse is showing clinical signs. A thorough questioning should include the groom, the rider, owner and, if during an event, contact should be established with the barn veterinarian at home. The through questioning will help to narrow down the enormous number of substances and toxins. However, if this does not provide enough evidence for a more limited group of suspects I would take the following samples: EDTA blood for a complete blood count and heparinized blood for a chemistry profile; a urine sample for immediate urine analysis. I strongly recommend collecting the following samples from the horse: urine (100 ml), plasma (minimum of 20 ml), feces, feed (any roughage and concentrate), bedding and drinking water (500 ml). All samples should be stored frozen at -20 °C. In cases when the horse died or was euthanized every effort should be made to convince the owner that the horse needs to be submitted for a full pathological examination.

Group 2 (summarized by Barrie Grant)

The fundamental approach to a diagnosis of a neurological condition is the same as for any organ system: a complete understanding of the history, a complete physical exam starting with obtaining the vital signs and then progressing to a neurological exam. By the time a neurological exam has been completed the examiner should be able to have a reasonable idea if the patient is in Group 1 or

Group 2, what laboratory tests would help confirm or rule out certain conditions and what imaging tests should be considered.

The basic equipment is usually found in any ambulatory vehicle of veterinarians doing an equine practice and this includes thermometer, stethoscope, ophthalmoscope, spinal needles (3.5 and 6 inches), and digital radiography. Although rarely needed rapid access to a board, pipe or metal splints to stabilize a paralyzed front or hind leg will provide stability to an injured leg, which calms both the patient and the client.

Neurological exams should be standardized for completeness, gaining case experience and to be able to communicate with consultants. Ataxia in North America is usually given a grade of 0 to 5 (Mayhew system). The characteristics of each grade are as follows:

- Grade 0: normal.
- Grade 1: minimal neurological deficits noted with normal gaits and requires manipulative tests (crossing legs, tail sways, tight circles, walking up and down hills, blind folding, backing, response to a dull object).
- Grade 2: mild abnormal gaits seen at a walk (walks like a patient that has been sedated) and more obvious response to the manipulative tests. Patients can be performing successfully but when asked they have trouble with lead changes, going down hills at a trot or gallop, stumble, are heavy on the fore hand, require a lot of leg to maintain propulsion, knuckle over when stopping and bunny hop behind when cantering, and drag hind toes a lot at a trot.
- Grade 3: easy to see at a walk, look like a drunken camel at a trot, very obvious at a canter but they do not fall.
- Grade 4: very ataxic – will fall especially in tight circles or backing. Usually will refuse to go any faster than a walk.
- Grade 5: recumbent – may not even be able to become sternal even with encouragement.

Specific conditions

Fractures

- Skull

  Fracture of the skull usually has an acute onset and a history of some form of trauma. A direct blow by a kick of an object such as a fence, pipe stock etc. Horses that fall over (flippers) backward and strike the top of the skull (external occipital protuberance) often have loss of consciousness with mild to severe seizures and hemorrhage from the external ear and /or Nares. If they are able to stand they are obviously at least Grade 3 ataxic with a head tilt (torticollis), strabismus (unilateral or bilateral), nystagmus. Many times they

are visually blind as the countercoup fracture associated with this trauma can either directly traumatize the optic nerve or the hemorrhage into the tight compartment in the Circle of Willis puts pressure on the optic nerve which results in dysfunction. The patient should be stabilized with mild sedation (avoid acepromazine as it will increase chances of seizure) anti- inflammatory medication (flunixin – 500mg /iv for 500 kg, dexamethasone 40 mg iv for 500 kg, and DMSO (200 ml diluted in 3 liters plasmalyte and given IV over a 2 hour period. An ophthalmologic exam will usually disclose a dilated pupil, lack of menace, normal eyelid tone and swelling of the optic nerve.
If the patient is stable then standing pharyngeal films will show the guttural pouch to be filled with fluid (hemorrhage) instead of air. Only rarely will the fracture at the symphysis of the basioccipital and sphenoid bone be noted, as the fractures are usually compression in nature. Endoscopy will show hemorrhage from the guttural pouch openings and even into the pharyngeal wall.
The prognosis depends on the response to time and anti-inflammatory medication. If there is still blindness after 30 days with a dilated pupil and atrophy of the optic disc the prognosis for performance is poor.
If the patient is recumbent and having seizures then anti- inflammatory medications are essential along with protection of the limbs and skull (especially the orbit and eyes) with extensive bandaging and use of protective hoods. It may be necessary to provide anesthesia to facilitate transportation to a facility equipped to deal with such a severe case. If after 8 to 12 hours of repeated sedation the seizures have not improved, the patient cannot stand even in a sling and they are a danger to themselves and handlers then euthanasia may have to be considered. I personally had a yearling colt that did not stand for 36 hours, required a sling for over 6 weeks and had marked truncal ataxia for a year. He did become a breeding stallion and was ranked 10th in the state of Washington.
Open fractures of the Cranial Vault are rare on patients that are still alive at the time of your initial exam. If this is the case the wounds need to be covered to reduce contamination and they need to be transported to a facility that can surgically debride the area and close the defects with the recovered pieces of bone or a sliding graft of the temporalis muscle and fascia. Aggressive antibiotic therapy needs to be started along with the above-mentioned anti-inflammatory therapy.

- Stylohyoid osteoarthropathy
  This condition has been one of the leading causes of sudden onset of seizures and ataxia in middle age to older horses at our referral hospital. Although the condition can be classified as a degenerative and chronic in nature there is often a traumatic episode (often cribbing) that fractures the degenerative bone and produces such acute pain and swelling seizures and facial nerve (VII) paralysis occur. With less severe forms the patient presents with a drooping and paralysis

of the affected ear and eyelid and lateral deviation of the nostril. There is often linear erosion or ulceration of the cornea from drying, as the eyelids do not fully close. They have a poor menace, decreased tone to the eyelid but will have a normal pupillary response to stimulus with a bright light. There is often pain to deep digital palpation over the temporo-mandibular joint and posterior mandible area. DV radiographs of the skull show a thickened stylohyoid bone and the lateral projection will often show a fracture callous. Endoscopy shows a thickened stylohyoid bone often with an increase in small vessels on the surface of the bone. If any question we always try to visualize the normal side. A nuclear imaging scan shows increased isotope activity at the petrous temple bone area. A CT scan is very definitive and can increase the clinician's ability to provide and accurate diagnosis and prognosis. Treatment consists of anti-inflammatory medication and surgical removal of the ceratohyoid bone. The surgery should be done early to afford the best chance to reduce the inflammation to the facial nerve. If delayed there is a good chance vision will be lost and the affected eye may have to be removed.

- Cervical spine
  Fractures of the cervical spine usually have history of trauma with an acute onset. Falling on the cervical area while jumping, pulling back when tied to an inanimate object or running into a stout fence with the head extended are characteristic histories. They may also present as colic as the pain and discomfort is very obvious. Foals with Salter fractures of the cervical body endplates have a dramatic ventral distortion of the midcervical area. If the patient is in lateral recumbence and cannot become sternal then a fracture of the lower cervical bodies with severe cord compression should be considered.
  Radiography is indicated to assist in the diagnosis. Initial treatment is the standard anti- inflammatory medications previously mentioned. They should be offered feed and water in an elevated (chest high) position. The degree of ataxia will improve rapidly in most cases. If the patient is still standing and radiographs show a fracture additional imaging such as CT scans and myelography are not indicated unless the degree of ataxia does not improve or becomes more dramatic. Often the articulation anterior or posterior to the fracture causes cervical stenosis. The majority of cases do improve and either return to competition or in the case of a foal develops into performance horses. I have repaired a linear fracture of the axis (C2) with lag screws.
  Only rarely will a neoplastic mass result in acute ataxia but we are reporting on two show horses (one Tb and one a Welsh pony) that stumbled and fell while jumping in competition that had space occupying neoplasm (a lymphoma and a hemangiosarcoma). Both patients had myelograms and surgical decompression but only the Tb with the lymphoma could be ridden safely again and that was only for a short period of time before the signs recurred.

- Thoracic spine

  Trauma to the thoracic spine is usually a result of falling over backwards and directly striking the dorsal spines or being trapped beneath very stout objects and trying to rise (a pipe restraining stock). Fractures of the dorsal spine usually are from T4- T8 and there is marked deformity (a flattened withers) and swelling. There is local pain and the patient does not want to move. If there is ataxia then a fracture of the body of the thoracic spine should be ruled out. Reasonable radiographs can be obtained of the majority of the bodies of the thoracic spines by using a technique for imaging the lungs. The air in the lungs produces a good contrast. Typically the fractures would be compressive so each segment needs to be measured to see if they are shorter in length. Treatment of the fractures of the summits of the spine should be conservative. Exploration of the fracture hematoma and removal of the fracture pieces is not indicated and often can lead to chronic infections and in one very notable case a descending infection into the spinal canal.

- Lumbar spine

  The lumbar spine (often the TL junction) can suffer catastrophic trauma especially if the animal has been traveling at a high velocity and trips and then summersaults and lands on the lumbar area. The majority of horses are unable to rise and many are found dead in a pasture a short distance from some object. It is important to recognize that a fracture in this area is a possibility and do not subject the patient to long process of dragging into an ambulance, transportation to hospital and possible slinging. Spinal fluid from a lumbosacral tap may be normal or bloody. Subarachnoid corticosteroids could be injected as an attempt to reduce swelling. The prognosis is very unfavorable.

- Sacrum/coccygeal

  Fracture in this area can occur from falling and sitting on their haunches, falling of one side on hard pavement or from stress fractures in young racehorses. These are painful injuries and many patients show bizarre behavior often kicking out when moved or trying to run away from what seems to them to be a very noxious stimulus when the fracture fragments move. They often have at least Grade 2/5 ataxia. The most consistent neurological deficit is that of a caudal equina syndrome with inability to defecate and micturate (often the bladder is overflowing and the urine dribbles out) and a very weak and flaccid tail. These clinical signs are very similar to the neurological form of Herpes and there can be some initial problems sorting out the diagnosis. A rectal exam should be performed not only to evacuate the rectum but also to check for rectal tone and to palpate the bladder and manually assist in the emptying of it. While doing the rectal the examiner should turn the palm dorsally to palpate for a firm enlargement on the ventral aspect of the sacrum. If this is suspected then a rectal ultrasound exam assists in determining the

character of the enlargement. If it is a fracture then the surface of the bone will not be smooth and the fluid will have the character of blood. A nuclear image with increased isotope uptake is very useful in confirming trauma as the most likely cause of the neurological deficits. Fluid from a lumbosacral tap can be normal or xanthrochromic.
Treatment consists of anti-inflammatory medication, stall restriction, sedation if showing violent activity when moving and evacuation of the rectum and drainage of the bladder 4 times a day. The clinical signs can persist for 6 to 8 months. Epidural steroids are also indicated and can be repeated 2 to 3 times. We have done surgical decompression on 3 cases with positive results.

Spinal stenosis

Many young, middle aged and older performance horses have either one of both articular facets of the caudal vertebra (C6/C7 is the most common) enlarged often from a developmental problem (OCD) but can also have had a fracture. They can perform well for years but suddenly a traumatic incident (falling, pulling back) will be the straw that breaks the camels back. The degree of ataxia depends on the extent of the pathology.

A complete neurological exam will often show that the signs are more obvious on one side. Standing radiographs will show an enlarged facet and an ultrasound exam will also demonstrate an enlarged facet with a roughened surface. Using the ultrasound to guide a needle to administer intra-articular steroids can be done to reduce the swelling of the inflamed joint capsule that is putting pressure on the spinal cord. Many horses show dramatic results and can perform soon after. The owners, trainer and riders need to be informed. If the degree of ataxia is Grade 2/5 plus then we recommend a myelogram before intra-articular therapy as a more accurate diagnosis and prognosis can be given. If there is dramatic cord compression then an anterior interbody fusion is indicated.

Peripheral nerve abnormalities

- Pectoral limb
  A. Suprascapular nerve: usually a history of a direct frontal blow (running into another horse coming the opposite direction). There is usually swelling at the point of the shoulder and as the limb goes into a weight bearing phase the scapulohumeral joint luxates laterally. Usually no creptice is heard or palpated. Radiographs should be acquired to rule out a fracture. Treatment consists of anti-inflammatory medications, stall restriction. Surgical decompression by cutting a notch out of the Scapula is not done as frequently now as there were some cases that suffered fractures of the scapula. Ultrasound guided drainage of any hematoma

and possibly a fasciotomy should be considered. Patients can return to training depending on the extent of trauma to the nerve.

B. Radial nerve: usually direct trauma from a kick or being forced to lie on the leg for an extended period of time (anesthesia or a traumatic accident with overturned vehicles). There is a firm and often-painful swelling over the humerus. If the motor branches to the triceps muscles are affected then the elbow is dropped and the patient cannot bear weight on the limb. Initially this can cause the patient and owners a great deal of anxiety. Intensive anti-inflammatory therapy should be started. Radiographs should be obtained to rule out fractures and an ultrasound exam should be done to drain any hematoma and disclose the most likely landmarks for a standing fasciotomy. If the elbow is dropped then bandaging and splinting is not indicated but if the limb can become weight bearing with the carpus extended then applying heavy bandages (Robert- Jones) and a splint (10 cm pvc plummers pipe cut in half) works well. The condition often improves dramatically in 48 hours.

- Pelvic limb

  Sciatic nerve: most often seen with fractures of the pelvis that involve the lesser sciatic notch. The unique stay apparatus in the horse usually prevents the characteristic dropped hock appearance seen in cats and dogs. The patients present with signs that mimic a peroneal nerve paralysis – that being dragging of the toes and inability to extend the toe. If the toe is extended then the patient can bear weight on the leg. It is important to rule out the source of the trauma to the nerve i.e. either from the lesser sciatic notch or trauma over the lateral aspect of the stifle. Radiographs of the stifle along with a rectal exam and ultrasound exam of the pelvis will help with the diagnosis. Treatment consists of anti-inflammatory medications, stall confinement and the application of a brace or splint of the lower limb to assist in keeping the toe extended. Without a brace and bandage severe ulcerated wounds of the dorsal aspect of the fetlock joint (and some with direct extension into the joint) will occur. The prognosis would have to be guarded as I have only one or two cases that I can recall to base any informed opinion on. But the patients cannot improve if they are dead.

Specific cases where physiotherapy made an improvement in equine sport

Christel Auer
Zur Dornermühle 60, 78224 Singen, Germany; ppt_team@yahoo.de

Introduction

Physiotherapy is the external application of therapeutic exercise and of therapeutic modalities. The goal of treatment is a natural, physiological reaction from the patient (for example: muscle growth, increased metabolism) intended to restore, preserve or facilitate normal function and development. Physiotherapy uses passive and active therapeutic modalities (forms of therapy) to prevent or heal medical conditions. This makes Physiotherapy an alternative or important component to conservative and operative treatments.

Some definitions

Structures of the body are parts of the body like organs, extremities and their specific parts. Body functions are the physiological functions of an organism including mental / psychological function. Damage / impairment are problems of structure of the body and body functions, like basic abnormalities, discrepancies, or loss of function.

Body functions

Classification of Body Functions (Quoted from 'International Classification of Functioning, Disability and Health ICF' approved by the World Health Assembly in May 2001)

- Mobility of joint function: range and ease of movement of a joint.
- Stability of joint function: maintenance of structural integrity of the joints.
- Muscle power function: force generated by the contraction of a muscle or muscle groups.
- Muscle tone function: tension present in the resting muscles and the resistance offered when trying to move the muscles passively.

Physiotherapeutic measures

Manual therapy

Manual therapy serves the purpose of discovering (diagnosing) and treating reversible losses of function to the musculoskeletal system. There are special handling techniques which serve, within the limits of medical findings, to localize and analyze reduced mobility and function in any particular joint (including the spinal column). The essential concept of manual therapy 'treatment with the use of the therapists hands' is thereby a small component of an extensive therapeutic concept.

Myofascial Trigger Point therapy

Trigger points are muscle fibres in which an inflammatory reaction exists with far reaching effects. Higher concentrations of specific neuropeptides have been found in painful trigger points and could be removed through the therapy. This information helps to explain the neurophysiology of trigger points and how they can cause the development of chronic, treatment-resistant pain.

Stretching

Even though the newest hypothesis suggest that stretching has no effect on performance, one should not forget that the elasticity of a muscle is together with strength, speed and endurance a factor of performance. Muscular disbalance and 'contractions' cannot be corrected through stretching. For such problems strengthening of the antagonists is indicated. Injury prevention is also not aided through stretching, as well as delayed onset muscle soreness (stretching actually tends to provoke this problem).

Proprioception

One can define the goal of proprioceptive training as to increase the ability of one's body to react better and more competently. The newest studies show that through proprioceptive training the risk of injury can be remarkably reduced. This modality aims at training the reflective muscle activity (through passive and active movement) as well as the restoration and stabilization of the structural integrity of the affected joints. How well proprioceptors can be trained is still uncharted territory as far as concrete studies go, only the functionality and adaptive capabilities of our nervous system are known. Evidence of adaptation is:

- increased networking and contact between specific cerebral areas;
- increased conductivity of the nerves due to a 'growing' myelin sheath (an insulating sheath which helps to forward impulses from nerve cell to nerve cell/nerve cell to other cells);
- an increase of the contact surface of the synapse;
- an increase in the support of heavily used synapse from lesser used ones.

Massage therapy

Pressure and tension have a mechanical effect on the layers of skin, fascia, muscle, tendon, joint capsule and connective tissue with their nerves, lymphatic and blood vessels. Scars and adhesions between tissues can be relieved through such mechanical effects.

Classic massage: a form of massage that deals mainly with treating muscle tissue. It has a relaxing and pain relieving effect, and also increases blood circulation as well as lymphatic circulation to the treated areas of the body.

Reflex zone therapy (Zone therapy, Reflexology): different forms of connective tissue massage, segmental massage, periosteal massage, and colon massage can be useful to influence positively inner organs. Through massaging reflex zones (skin-nerve-areas) a therapist influences the tension surrounding inner organs reducing pain in those areas.

Manual lymphatic drainage: through specialized gentle massage techniques, a therapist can cause the lymphatic ducts (as well as the veins in the area) to open up (dilate) and drain. Swelling due to injury or surgery as well as rheumatic disorders, can be successfully treated through manual lymphatic drainage. This treatment often reduces pain.

Thermotherapy

Heat therapy involves radiation (for example infrared light) or conduction to create warmth:

- sauna;
- 'hot roll': hot water poured into a tightly rolled up towel, carefully applied over the region to be treated;
- ultrasound to increase metabolism and relieve adhesions;
- peloids.

Cryotherapy is treatment using low temperature in the form of:

- crushed ice mixed with salt water or ice packed in towels frozen in salt water;
- conventional ice packs;
- ice massage: the direct application of ice to the skin, performed by rubbing the ice in a circular, massaging motion;
- cryogenic chamber therapy, cold air treatment.

Warmth reduces pain, increases circulation and metabolism. It relaxes the muscles and improves the elasticity of the connective tissue. Also not to be forgotten is the calming effect on the vegetative system.

The ultrasonic waves create a mechanical effect to treated areas through vibration. Pain reduction, increased circulation and metabolism, as well as muscle relaxation are the results. Adhesions can also be relieved through ultrasonic therapy.

Cold leads to a short term increase in the tension of a muscle. Cold application can stop pain through a decrease in nerve conductivity and curbing the pain receptors (nociceptors).

Hydrotherapy

Hydrotherapy is the application of cold and warm water. This can be done 1) by spouting water on a region of the body for example the lower leg, usually starting with warm water, then cold, always beginning at the farthest point away from the heart and then working towards the heart, and 2) with packs: the patient is wrapped in warm or cold dampened sheets, meant to either draw heat, conserve heat or provoke perspiration. For additional effects one can add clay, curd or specific plant substances (like extracts) to the packs.

Electrotherapy

To date, there is little 'research' data (on the basis of *random, controlled* clinical testing) on the effects of electrotherapy. Many patients have experienced the benefits of the therapeutic modalities. However, the practical physiotherapist lacks the resources to prove the effects in a clinical situation (in terms of evidence based medicine).

Galvanized current: through the application of electrical current between a positive and negative charged electrode, a therapist can achieve pain reduction as well as increased circulation and metabolism in the treated tissues creating optimal healing circumstances.

Low frequency current (0-1000 Hz): provokes nerves and muscles to contract. Good for use in preventing atrophied muscles and to aid in the recovery after partial paralysis.

Middle frequency current / Interfering current (1-100 Hz): depending on the form of application it will produce pain reduction or stimulate muscle stimulation followed by relaxation. One can also use this form of electrotherapy to increase circulation and reduce swelling.

The application of physiotherapy in equine sports

I would like to share with you the following publication released from the German Olympic Sports Committee and would like to ask you to read 'horse' when 'athlete' is mentioned.

> **Sports medicine examination and supervision system**
>
> Since 1970, every national athlete has the possibility to undergo for free (paid by the state) a yearly assessment. The goals are:
> - to determine the status and conservation of an athletes general health;
> - to determine the athletes capacity to compete;
> - to maintain adequate performance levels through early diagnosis and treatment of decreased function and injuries;
> - to prevent sport related decrease in the further wellbeing of the athletes.
>
> The on site treatment and supervision of athletes through board certified specialists in Sports Medicine and by Sport Physiotherapists has the following goals:
> - to prevent discipline specific micro-traumas and further deterioration;
> - to conserve an athletes capacity at the optimal training intensity;
> - to eliminate weaknesses that can later have effects on the musculoskeletal system;
> - to introduce newest knowledge on prevention, regeneration and treatment into top level sports;
> - to apply the latest methods in the training. Performance diagnosis has to be done by or under supervision by a Doctor of Sports Medicine.
>
> The supervision of athletes by sport medicine professionals means daily control of the exercise to prevent injuries, assess the athletes capacity to train and regenerate (including explaining the risks of doping). The supervision can be done by an Olympic Committee doctor, a sport association doctor, or a sport physiotherapist.

When I read these points, I realize that few riders consider that their high performance athletes need support. The application of physiotherapy should be, as in human sports, an integral part of performance conservation and improvement in equine sports, and not a fashion. Physiotherapy will find its place in equine sports. The prerequisites are an exact definition of goals as well as the creation of a therapeutic modality to be integrated in the daily exercise plan of each horse based on individual needs.

The requirements to define clear physiotherapeutic goals in equine sports seem somewhat difficult because riders as well as veterinarians lack understanding on how physiotherapy can be of benefit. It would be beneficial for the veterinarians to learn about what sort of impact physiotherapy can have. They should work with a physiotherapist. For the rider it must be clear that physiotherapy does not replace good riding and training. Physiotherapy can help the organism to perform its best only with continuous application. Until now in most cases the rider will first seek the help of a physiotherapist when a severe drop in performance takes place, sometime shortly before a big event or even at the event. Physiotherapy may help in these situations but prevention is much more effective.

Some typical cases

Case 1

It is the weekend before the 5-year-old dressage championships to take place on Wednesday. Sunday afternoon the horse stands in the arena stiff as a board and does not respond to the commands to move forward. Every trick fails. Even when the horse is led it moves stiff and uncomfortably. My assumption was that the horse was exercised so much beyond capacity that it simply could not go on. By palpation the horse reacted to the slightest touch in a painful manner.

Course of therapy

- Sunday: cold water spouting on the leg and a classic massage to loosen up the sore muscles.
- Monday morning: magnetic field therapy, walking in almost shoulder deep cold water for ten minutes, manual lymphatic drainage.
- Monday afternoon: physiotherapeutic treatment (massage, trigger point therapy, and proprioceptive training).
- Monday evening: magnetic field therapy, blanketed with a light wool blanket.
- Tuesday morning: magnetic field therapy, walking in cold water for 20 minutes, light riding, physiotherapeutic treatment
- Tuesday afternoon: transport to event.
- Tuesday evening: light riding, magnetic field therapy, lightly blanketed afterwards.
- Wednesday morning: magnetic field therapy, physiotherapeutic treatment, light riding.
- Wednesday afternoon: placed in the top six.

Case 2

Under the threat of not making the team for the World Championships the horse seems to suffer a total performance collapse. The horse is unusually stressed, refuses to take weight on his hind quarters, does not carry the bit, carries his head high above the withers creating an unwanted extension in the spinal cord causing him to loose his timing in the trot. As I observed the horses posture I realized that his back was sunken, his hind end standing far back, his abdominal muscles appeared weak and his back muscle was extremely tense and sunken where the saddle would go. The horse was extremely sensitive to be touched and the muscles hard and non-elastic through most of the body. There were no blockades of joints based on my chiropractic examination. In a person I would have suspected a burn-out syndrome accompanied by spastic muscles and massive appearance of trigger-points.

Course of therapy

- Daily: magnetic field therapy morning and evening
- Week 1: three times per week physiotherapeutic treatment, ultrasonic therapy, light bascule oriented riding, hacking, paddock twice a day for an hour.
- Week 2: two times per week physiotherapeutic treatment, cranio-sacral treatment once, two times light flatwork with emphasis on the cool down phases, careful of fatigue, hacking, paddock once a day for an hour.
- Week 3: two times per week physiotherapeutic treatment, cranio-sacral treatment once, three times light flatwork with emphasis on the cool down phases, hacking, paddock once a day for an hour.
- Week 4 and 5: physiotherapeutic treatment once, cranio-sacral treatment once, reintroduction of the normal training program with emphasis on the cool down phases, hacking, paddock once a day for an hour
- Week 6: physiotherapeutic treatment once, normal training program. Examination and therapeutic supervision at the competition; drastic performance improvement.
- Week 7: physiotherapeutic treatment once, back to Grand Prix oriented training. Examination and therapeutic supervision at the competition.

At the World Championships the horse developed a massive stress colic. The team vet allowed the horse to be treated conservatively, therapist supervision the entire time, after two hours normal gastric noises, somewhat tense muscles that through the above mentioned techniques were loosened, manual lymphatic drainage. Horse performed for the national team.

Since the world championships I have been treating the horse successfully once every two to three weeks.

Case 3

During an international competition a horse had a large loss of performance: looses its form over the fence, will not open up over the oxers and runs away after landing. 28 faults on the first day. After a short examination I find that his entire back muscles are tense and sore to the touch, his lumbar region is hard as a rock. The M. iliocostalis lumborum is extremely sensitive, flexing and lateral bending is not possible.

Course of therapy

- Day 1: hot roll, classic massage and trigger point therapy in his lumbar region, M. iliocostalis lumborum as well as M. obliquus externus between his last two ribs and tuber coxae; magnetic field therapy.
- Day 2
  - Morning: magnetic field therapy, classic massage, mobilization of the horse in form of walking.
  - Afternoon: magnetic field therapy once more, no faults and into the jump off for the national team.
  - Evening: hot roll with a classic massage and magnetic field therapy.

For the horses well-being he got the weekend off.

Case 4

Finally, I would like to talk about my best teacher 'Excellent'. His rider came to me in 1996 and said that he had a problem with his horse: 'He is so hard in his mouth during the course, fights against the bit, is stiff in his ribs and no longer opens up over the oxers'. Excellent gave the impression of being very stiff under his rider. I realized that by palpation he would hold his breath and contract his muscles. The space between his ribs was very stiff and the ribs themselves showed no mobility. I tried every therapeutic modality and technique. He received therapy every two weeks. It was amazing and fascinating to watch and *feel* how he reacted to each treatment and technique. Nowadays he shows no pain and responds adequately to all commands. Excellent has been under my therapeutic supervision since and I still learn something new from him every time I treat him. He is also the first horse that I accompanied to important events and I treated him at the following tournaments:

- 1997 European Championships in Mannheim;
- 1998 World Championships in Rom;
- 1999 European Championships in Hickstead;
- 2000 Olympic Games in Sydney;

- Until 2003 many international competitions under the riding of Samantha McIntosh;
- Starting mid 2003 under the riding of Alexander Auer; victory in Finals of the Baden Wurttemburg Championships of Young Riders – Silver Medal;
- 2004 Top 10 in the Baden Wurttemburg Championships, many international Placings in the category S;
- 2005 many wins in the category S;
- 2006 win in the mini Prix at the CSI Ravensburg;
- 2007 a season of rest;
- 2008 22 years young ridden by Christina Störk, placings in the category L.

At this point I would like to give my heartfelt thanks to his rider who knows from experience that physiotherapy can be extremely beneficial when consequently and regularly applied. When constantly supported an athlete can perform at top level for longer than one who does not receive the proper care and support that a top athlete requires. Physiotherapy is an integral part of the training of a top sport horse.

Sources of information

Deutscher Verband für Physiotherapie - Zentralverband der Physiotherapeuten/ Krankengymnasten (ZVK) e. V. Deutzer Freiheit 72-74, D-50679 Cologne; Germany; www.zvk.org/.

IGTM - Internationale Gesellschaft für Schmerz- und Triggerpunktmedizin e.V. Aufsessplatz 19, D-90456 Nuremberg, Germany; www.igtm.org/.

Dry Needling Verband Schweiz, Merkurstrasse 12; CH-8400 Winterthur, Switzerland; www.triggerpunkt-therapie.ch.

Verband Physikalische Therapie, Bundesgeschäftsstelle, Hofweg 15, D-22085 Hamburg; Germany; www.vpt-online.de.

Poor performance: could it be caused by respiratory malfunction?

Marianne M. Sloet van Oldruitenborgh-Oosterbaan[1] and J.Geoffrey Lane[2]
[1]Department of Equine Sciences, Faculty of Veterinary Medicine, Utrecht University, Utrecht, the Netherlands; m.sloet@uu.nl
[2]Cedars Surgical Services, The Cedars, Cross, Axbridge, Somerset, BS26 2EG, United Kingdom; jgeoffreylane@gmail.com

Introduction

Abnormal noise (stridor) is generally taken to be a reliable presenting sign of poor performance attributable to respiratory impediments in athletic horses. There is a widely held belief amongst riders and owners that whenever an untoward noise is heard, particularly if it is inspiratory, the horse must be diseased and that optimal performance cannot be achieved. Conversely, they believe that the horse must be normal if no noises are heard. This contribution examines whether such relationships exist as well as discussing the potential causes of functional obstructions in the upper respiratory tract of the horse. At the outset it must be accepted that the measurement of performance, and by extension that of performance-limitation, is challenging even in sports such as racing where data on the performance records of each individual are available. Less detailed data are available for sports horses engaged in show jumping, dressage and eventing.

An inability to breathe freely provokes obvious performance-limitations for the athletic horse and the presenting signs in afflicted animals include reduced stamina through an inability to sustain aerobic muscle function and audible respiratory noises through increased turbulence within the upper respiratory tract. The minute volume of normal horses at rest is of the order of 80 l but this is increased to as much as 2500 l during fast exercise in racehorses. The pressure gradients required to move such large volumes of air can be as much as 40 cm water and these act across the walls of the airway so that considerable 'collapsing forces' come into play during inspiration. In the nasal passages and the trachea the semi-rigid structures lining the airway help to resist this effect but obvious areas of weakness lie at the nares and in the pharynx and larynx. At rest 70-85% of the total airway resistance arises at these points but through muscular effort this is reduced to approximately 50% during forced breathing. For example, the action of the naso-labialis muscles dilates the nares, the pharyngeal and intrinsic palatal musculature helps to maintain the patency of the musculo-membranous tube of the nasopharynx and the crico-arytenoideus dorsalis muscles abduct the cartilages of the larynx. Obviously there will be occasions when a structural deformity leads to compromised airflow, for example with intra-nasal masses, epiglottal entrapment, sub-epiglottal cysts and arytenoid chondropathy, but it is a failure to withstand the collapsing forces of respiration which is responsible whenever horses show signs of dynamic obstructive dyspnoea.

The limitations of endoscopic examinations made during quiet breathing, i.e. when the patient is standing in the stable or has recently returned from exercise, are obvious and yet they form the lynch-pin of respiratory investigations for most veterinarians in equine clinical practice. The best means to achieve a definitive diagnosis of dynamic airway obstructions is to assess the patient while it is exercising vigorously and endoscopy during highspeed treadmill exercise has been the gold standard technique for the past two decades. The advantages and limitations of overground endoscopes have yet to be documented.

Although the spectrum of disorders that can cause dynamic airway obstruction in the upper respiratory tract is similar within the different breeds the significance varies greatly in parallel with the exertion required across the range of equine athletic activities. In Warmblood horses recurrent laryngeal neuropathy is probably the most common cause whereas in Thoroughbreds and Standardbreds dorsal displacement of the soft palate and palatal instability are more common.

Compromised exercise capacity of the equine athlete is of great importance and a complete clinical and endoscopic examination at rest and at exercise is necessary to diagnose or to eliminate upper respiratory tract malfunction as the cause.

Clinical examination

Although this aspect is often overlooked, an examination starts with taking an accurate history of the horse. For the tentative diagnosis of upper airway problems it is important to ask:

- What is the exact complaint of the horse?
- What was the duration and progress of the complaint?
- If there is a noise: does the noise wax and wane, is it present throughout exercise, or does it only arise under extreme exertion?
- Does the sound change with speed and/or head position?
- How long has the owner/rider/trainer had the horse?
- Was the problem present at the time of purchase or did it develop subsequently?
- Does the performance record of the horse suggest that it has deteriorated or is this an animal with an inherent lack of ability?

Physical examination should be done at rest and after exercise. At rest the breathing pattern, the effort and the rate should be noted. In most cases of respiratory noise and/or dynamic obstruction of the upper respiratory tract, no abnormalities will be found at rest. Airflow at the nostrils should be equal. If a nasal discharge is present, the type of discharge should be noted and also whether it is unilateral or bilateral and whether discharge is only seen under certain conditions. A foul smell may be indicative for tissue necrosis, certain infections or neoplasia. The head and neck should be carefully inspected with regard to general attitude and expression, facial asymmetry and cranial nerve dysfunction, nostril width and nasal drainage.

After inspection the head and neck are palpated in detail. The nasal passages, false nostrils, thickness of the nasal septum, width of the intermandibular space are checked. Palpation of the larynx for asymmetry is very useful in the Thoroughbred but sometimes more difficult in the heavier Warmblood horses. The diagnosis of the 4th branchial arch defect (4-BAD) syndrome is especially based on a thorough palpation. Laryngeal palpation should establish whether the cartilage skeleton is complete or defective, whether there is a detectable atrophy of the intrinsic musculature and whether there is a ventral or lateral cicatrix indicative of previous surgery. The trachea has to be palpated for anomalies such as fractured or irregular tracheal rings or scars from earlier surgery. During the whole physical examination one should be alert on signs of previous surgery of head and neck.

Endoscopic examination

Endoscopic examination of the upper respiratory tract provides a ready diagnosis of most diseases that cause abnormal noise resulting from structural changes. Additional information can be obtained by partial nostril occlusion to stimulate an increased amplitude of laryngeal abductor movement and flushing water through the endoscope to stimulate swallowing. For a complete examination at rest, both nasal meati and ethmoturbinates, the nasopharynx, larynx and trachea are carefully examined.

For a standardized digital video clip for the KWPN stallion examination it is necessary to:

- Provide requested information about identification, age and date of examination of the DVD.
- Examine the horse at rest with a twitch; if a sedative is necessary this should be indicated clearly with name of drug, dose and time before endoscopy.
- Pass endoscope through right nostril and film the larynx at rest during 30 seconds.
- Continue filming while inducing movement of the larynx through occlusion of both nostrils (at least 1x full adduction and 1x full abduction); then, perform 'slap-test' behind the left shoulder twice.

- If the larynx is not fully symmetrical the procedure has to be repeated completely through the left nostril; now the slap-test should be performed twice behind the right shoulder.

In many horses with stridor or decreased performance resulting from upper airway disorders, the endoscopy at rest reveals no abnormality and endoscopy during highspeed treadmill exercise is indicated. Depending on the individual horse and the preference of the clinician one to five schooling sessions are necessary before the procedure is performed. Occasionally horses are found to be temperamentally unsuitable and cannot be examined. Some clinicians prefer to perform the treadmill endoscopy with a simple snaffle bridle and some prefer a head collar only.

After a warm-up the endoscope is passed via the right or left nostril and the distal tip is positioned within the nasopharynx at the level of the openings of the auditory tube diverticula. This position allows a clear view of the larynx and the caudal portion of the nasopharynx and soft palate. The endoscope can be secured to the noseband of the head collar using a length of latex rubber tubing and a bulldog clip or using a specially made cotton strap with adjustable Velcro strip. During exercise any abnormal respiratory sound should be noticed.

Endoscopic abnormalities observable at rest

Nasal passage abnormalities

Examples in this group are:

- Progressive ethmoidal haematoma – slowly expanding angiomatous masses that most likely originate from the mucosal lining of ethmoturbinates either on the sinus or nasal aspect. PEH's occasional cause nasal noise before epistaxis is observed.
- Sinu-nasal cysts are more common than PEH and may cause nasal obstruction.
- Atheroma – aberrant epithelial tissue remaining after embryogenesis and causing unilaterally a cyst-like anomaly in the false nostril.
- Alar fold obstruction – alar folds are drawn into the nasal passage during inspiration producing a loud vibrating nasal noise.
- Congenital nasal septal cysts, septal deviations, neoplastic infiltration, amyloid disposition, nasal polyps and nasal septum cartilage degeneration are rare.
- Fungal granulomas of the nasal passage – rare in Western European countries.

Pharyngeal lymphoid hyperplasia

This is also known as follicular pharyngitis or lymphoid follicular hyperplasia. This enlargement of the pharyngeal lymphoid follicles is frequently observed in young horses and is considered to be a normal physiological finding.

Nasopharyngeal cicatrix

This abnormality is characterised by a structuring web of tissue in the wall of the nasopharynx. The disorder has only been reported from North America and usually arises concurrent with arytenoid chondropathy.

Chondritis of the arytenoid cartilages

Microabscess formation within the cartilage matrix of one or both arytenoids. The aetiopathogenesis is not known but the condition leads to dystrophic changes, including enlargement, axial displacement, inflammation and reduced motility by the diseased cartilage. As the disease progresses granulation tissue may project from the surface or there may be changes in the shape of the arytenoid cartilage with restriction of the rima glottidis. Contact ulcers of the mucous membrane of the contra-lateral arytenoid may be present. The presence and extent of mineralisation of affected tissues can be evaluated on a lateral radiograph.

Epiglottic entrapment (EE)

Epiglottic entrapment is characterised by envelopment of the apex of the epiglottis and its margins by sub-epiglottic mucosa and the ary-epiglottic folds. Some entrapments are unstable and may only be intermittently visible. Repeated stimulation to swallow should be a routine component of all endoscopic examinations in order to give the best opportunity to identify an entrapment. Under exercise conditions EE may cause a wide range of abnormal inspiratory and expiratory noises and may also provoke secondary DDSP.

Pharyngeal cysts

Pharyngeal cysts are fluid filled round structures that occur most commonly in the sub-epiglottic region but may occur within the soft palate and on the dorsal wall of the nasopharynx. Often sub-epiglottic cysts move from the nasopharynx to the oro-pharynx during swallowing and to make such cysts visible it is important that the horse swallows several times during the examination. Additionally a radiograph of the laryngeal and pharyngeal area may help in the diagnosis.

Neoplasia of the nasopharynx

The tentative diagnosis of neoplasia in the nasopharynx is based on visible aberrant tissue formation. The most frequent neoplasia arising at this site are lymphosarcoma and squamous cell carcinoma.

Recurrent laryngeal neuropathy (RLN)

Recurrent laryngeal neuropathy or idiopathic laryngeal hemiplegia is paresis or paralysis of the left vocal fold as result of degeneration of the axons in the recurrent laryngeal nerve supplying the larynx.

There are a number of different schemes to grade laryngeal function. Whatever method is used it must have consistency so that it is repeatable for the clinician. Some veterinarians prefer to give an actual description in words of the arytenoid symmetry, movement and response to slap-test, because an individual horse can have significant observable alterations in laryngeal symmetry and movement over variable periods of time; sometimes better and sometimes worse. The best way to determine the clinical significance of varying degrees of recurrent laryngeal neuropathy is endoscopy during high-speed treadmill exercise.

Endoscopic abnormalities only observed during exercise

Arytenoid cartilage collapse (ACC)

ACC is a dynamic movement of the corniculate process of the arytenoid cartilage towards the midline of the rima glottidis during inspiration, resulting in severe narrowing of the laryngeal airway. This is invariably accompanied by ipsilateral vocal cord collapse, except in cases where the vocal cord had been removed during previous surgery. ACC can be partial and may not accompanied by vocal cord collapse. ACC is invariably accompanied by an inspiratory noise.

Vocal cord collapse (VCC)

VCC is a dynamic collapse of one (unilateral) or both (bilateral) vocal folds towards the midline during inspiration resulting in a bowed configuration of the cord(s) which would normally be seen as straight and tense. VCC is invariably accompanied by an inspiratory noise.

Axial deviation of the ary-epiglottic folds (ADAF)

ADAF is a medial displacement of the vertical margins of the ary-epiglottic folds. Rarely it may occur as the sole cause of dynamic airway obstruction but much more frequently it arises concurrent with one or more other forms of dynamic collapse typically palatal malfunction. Harsh inspiratory sounds are usually heard in horses with ADAF where the volume of the noise is related to the severity of the axial displacement.

Palatal instability (PI)

PI is progressive dorso-ventral billowing movements of particularly the caudal portion of the soft palate with flattening of the ventral surface of the epiglottis against the dorsal surface of the soft palate. The billowing waves may commence rostrally and ponies are particularly prone to rostral billowing of the soft palate. Rough inspiratory and expiratory noises typically accompany PI but some PI is silent to the unaided ear.

Dorsal displacement of the soft palate (DDSP)

During DDSP the caudal border of the soft palate moves to a position above the epiglottis during high intensity exercise and remains displaced through a variable number of respiratory cycles until it is restored to its normal position by swallowing. DDSP is always preceded by PI but not all PI leads on to DDSP. Contrary to previous reports DDSP is never a sequel to deglutition. Repeated cycles of DDSP and replacement may be seen until the exercise test is completed. Vibrant predominantly expiratory noises, sometimes termed 'choking' or 'gurgling' typically accompany DDSP but, again, some DDSP is silent to the unaided ear.

Conclusion

There is a tendency in clinical practice to make simple single diagnoses but treadmill endoscopy has shown that dynamic collapse in the equine upper respiratory tract is often complex with multiple sources of obstruction. On the other hand the traditional assumption that RLN and DDSP often go together holds some water – over 40% of horses with collapse of the arytenoid cartilage and / or vocal fold show concurrent palatal malfunction – DDSP or PI.

Clearly not all horses which show poor or deteriorating performance and/or which make untoward respiratory noises at exercise can be referred for highspeed treadmill endoscopy. The selection of horses for this technique should include those patients where the noises heard at exercise cannot be explained by the findings of palpation or endoscopy; horses which fade abruptly in races without abnormal respiratory sounds; and horses where previous airway surgery has been unsuccessful. For veterinary surgeons in equine clinical practice endoscopy during quiet breathing has become the primary technique for the diagnosis of obstructive disorders of the URT and yet, there is now a wealth of evidence to show that when performed in isolation this technique is unreliable. In an ideal world all equine athletes with perceived poor performance, particularly those exhibiting signs of upper respiratory tract obstruction, would be evaluated by highspeed treadmill endoscopy. The primary objection to this philosophy may be based on financial considerations and yet, owners, trainers and their veterinary advisors may be guilty of misguided economic restraint. The losses sustained as a result of incomplete or incorrect diagnoses may be considerable. Not only should the cost of inappropriate treatments be taken into consideration, but to this should be added the costs of convalescence, futile training, additional surgeries, loss of earnings and patient devaluation.

Suggested reading

Frankin, S.H., J.R. Naylor and J.G. Lane, 2006. Video-endoscopic evaluation of the upper respiratory tract in 93 sport horses during exercise testing on a high-speed treadmill. Equine vet. J. (2006) Suppl. 36: 540-545.

Lane, J.G., B. Bladon, D.R.M. Little, J.R.J. Naylor and S.H. Franklin, 2008A. Dynamic obstructions of the equine upper respiratory tract. Part 1: Observations during high-speed treadmill endoscopy of 600 Thoroughbred racehorses. Equine vet. J. 38: 393-399.

Lane, J.G., B. Bladon, D.R.M. Little, J.R.J. Naylor and S.H. Franklin, 2008B. Dynamic obstructions of the equine upper respiratory tract. Part 2: Comparison of endoscopic findings at rest and during high-speed exercise of 600 Thoroughbred racehorses. Equine vet. J. 38: 401-408.

Lane, J.G., 2007. Fourth branchial arch defects. In: Equine respiratory medicine and surgery. Eds. McGorum BC, Dixon, PM, Robinson NE and Schumacher J. Saunders Elsevier, Edinburgh, pp. 467-472.

Sloet van Oldruitenborgh-Oosterbaan, M.M., 1996. Review of respiratory noises ('Kehlkopfpfeifen') in the horse. Pferdeheilkunde 12: 698-702.

Sloet van Oldruitenborgh-Oosterbaan, M.M., 2005. How do breeding programme restrictions influence the incidence of recurrent laryngeal neuropathy? Third World Equine Airways Symposium. http://www.ivis.org/proceedings/WEAS/2005/Sloet/chapter.asp?LA=1.

Abstracts

Effect of forage: concentrate ratio on acid-base balance and racing performance

D.E. Allen[1], J.M. Ellis[1], R.G. Wilkinson[2], T. Carey[1] and T. Hollands[3]
[1]Warwickshire College, Moreton Morrell, Warwickshire, United Kingdom
[2]Harper Adams University College, Newport, Shropshire, United Kingdom
[3]Dodson and Horrell LTD, Islip, Kettering, Northants, United Kingdom

Take home message

Forage:concentrate ratio has significant effects on racehorse acid-base metabolism and performance with the effects of a high oat ration appearing to be more detrimental than a high compound feed ration.

Introduction

The horse evolved to survive on rations high in forage. Most racehorses are fed rations containing reduced levels of forage, with a corresponding increase in concentrate supply. Such forage reductions are widely established to be associated with a corresponding number of physiological and psychological adaptations. Gastrointestinal tract disorders such as colic (Tinker *et al.*, 1997), metabolic disorders such as exertional rhabdomyolysis (Macleay *et al.*, 2000), gastric ulcers (Cirelli 1993), laminitis (McLean *et al.*, 1998) and oral sterotypies such as crib biting (Willard *et al.*, 1977) are all associated with a reduction in forage intake.

Many of these problems are associated with alterations in the body's acid-base homeostasis. Such alterations are likely to occur due to the high starch and low dietary cation-anion levels associated with concentrate feedstuffs. This study investigates the nature and extent of the effects of reducing dietary roughage levels, whilst concurrently increasing dietary concentrate supply, on the acid base status and performance of the Thoroughbred racehorse.

Methods and materials

The protocol used in this trial was subject to the review and approval of the research committee of Warwickshire College.

Four thoroughbred type horses (two mares, one gelding and one stallion) aged 6.3 ± 3.6 years and weighing 550 ± 71 kg were used for this study. All horses had been adapted to a high-speed treadmill prior to the study.

The horses received four diets (80% forage: 20% concentrate [80H]; 50% forage: 50% concentrate [50H]; 30% forage: 70% concentrate (race mix) [30HM] and 30% forage: 70% concentrate (whole oats) [30HO] in a 4 x 4 Latin –square design. The diets consisted of forage in the form of haylage, and concentrate in the form of a racing coarse mix formulated for racing Thoroughbreds and horses in hard work, containing essential amino acids, vitamins and minerals, or whole oats. Each period of the trial consisted of fourteen days adaptation followed by a seven-day collection period.

The horses were exercised for one hour every day on a mechanical horse walker except days 2, 4, 9, 11 and 16 when the horses were exercised on the high-speed horse treadmill at walk, trot and gallop. On the seventh day of each collection period the horses were subjected to a maximal fatigue (adapted from that used by Eaton *et al.*, 1995) test on the high-speed treadmill. The test was continued until the handlers decided that an individual could no longer maintain the speed despite encouragement.

Urine pH, faecal pH, starch digestibility were measured throughout the trial. Time and distance traveled at fatigue, speed at fatigue, maximum heart rate, 1 minute recovery heart rate, and rectal temperature rise were recorded for each fatigue test. All data were subjected to analysis of variance to determine the significant difference between individuals and treatment using Genstat version 8.

Results

Mean ± SE urine pH was significantly ($P<0.001$) lower for the 30HM and 30HO diets compared to the 80H ration (7.27, 6.74 and 8.63 respectively).

Mean ± SE faecal pH was significantly ($P<0.001$) lower on the 30HM and 30HO diets compared to the 80H ration (7.03, 6.09 and 7.87 respectively).

Mean ± SE starch digestibility did not vary significantly with diet fed.

Mean ± SE speed at fatigue and distance traveled at fatigue were significantly ($P<0.05$) higher on the 30HM and 30HO diets compared to the 80H ration (11.4, 11.1 and 10.5 m/s and 6401.3, 6214.0 and 4914.5 m respectively). Mean ± SE time at fatigue, maximum heart rate, 1 minute recovery heart rate and rectal temperature rise were higher on the 30HM and 30HO diets compared to the 80H ration (920.75, 839.75 and 770.25 seconds, 192, 197 and 175 bpm, 135, 137 and 118 bpm, and 2.03, 2.35 and 1.83 °C respectively) although these effects were not significant.

Discussion and conclusion

This study investigated the effects of forage:concentrate ratios on acid-base status and racing performance. The two low forage diets (30HM, 30HO) were designed to reflect the most common rations fed within UK racing (Harris, 1999).

The diets, whilst varying in forage:concentrate ratio, also varied in DCAB, with the 80H diet being 399 mequiv/kg DM, and the 30HO diet being 221 mequiv/kg DM. The starch content ranged from 241.7 g/kg DM to 654 g/kg DM for the 80H and 30HO diets respectively. The effects of DCAB on the subjects were ascertained by measurement of urine pH (Zeyner *et al.*, 2002) whilst the affects of dietary starch content were ascertained by measurement of starch digestibility and faecal pH (Zeyner *et al.*, 2002). The effects of forage:concentrate ratio and acid-base status on racing performance were determined by use of a maximal fatigue test designed to reflect racing effort.

As forage intake decreased, DCAB decreased and urine pH significantly decreased ($P<0.001$). These findings are in line with those of Baker *et al.* (1992). Metabolically a low DCAB ration leads to metabolic acidosis and in order to maintain acid base homeostasis the kidney removes an increased concentration of hydrogen ions in the urine leading to reduced urine pH. (Tucker *et al.*, 1988). The urine acidity observed in the present study could potentially have significant impacts on other areas of metabolism, such as bone metabolism (Glade, 1983; Jackson *et al.*, 2001).

As forage intake decreased, starch intake increased and faecal pH significantly decreased ($P<0.001$). Starch digestibility remained relatively constant, irrespective of diet, and was found not to vary significantly ($P>0.05$) with diet. The horse is known to have a low amylase activity in the gastrointestinal tract in comparison to other species (Radicke *et al.*, 1992). As a consequence it has been suggested that on high starch diets the horse may digest a large proportion of starch by microbial fermentation within the large intestine (Radicke *et al.*, 1992; Kienzle, 1994). This results in the production of large concentrations of lactic acid (Garner *et al.*, 1977; Radicke *et al.*, 1992; Kienzle, 1994) leading to caecal acidosis and a reduction in faecal pH. These observations are in line with the findings of the present study whereby the total digestive tract starch digestibility remained relatively constant across the diets tested, however faecal pH was found to decrease from 7.87 on the 80H ration to 7.03 and 6.09 for the 30HM and 30HO diets respectively. This indicates the horses in the present study were digesting the high levels of dietary starch, caused by a reduction in forage intake, by using microbial digestion in the large intestine. Potentially this could have a large health and welfare impact on the horses concerned. Large intestine acidosis has been implicated as a potential cause of oral stereotypies (Willard *et al.*, 1997), laminitis (Garner *et al.*, 1977) and colic (Tinker *et al.*, 1997).

Time, distance traveled and speed at fatigue, heart rate during and post fatigue test, and rectal temperature rise during fatigue test, were used as parameters to indicate the effect of forage:concentrate ratio on racing performance. Results indicate that as forage intake is reduced, leading to a corresponding reduction in DCAB and an increase in starch intake, horses were able to gallop faster ($P<0.05$), further ($P<0.05$) and longer ($P>0.05$). This indicates better racing performance on a low forage: high concentrate diet, the effects were most marked where racing mix was used as the concentrate as opposed to whole oats. This is likely to be due to the more marked effects that the whole oats were seen to have on acid-base metabolism. Previous studies have indicated that low DCAB rations may have a significant impairment on performance (Graham-Thiers *et al.*, 1999). Whilst racing performance was improved in the present study, the heart rate and rectal temperature data indicate that the horses on the 30% forage diets were not working significantly harder than those on the 80% forage diets. This data may potentially indicate that high concentrate diets are advantageous to racing performance, probably due to their ability to supply glucose, the preferred energy substrate for maximal short duration exercise, such as that undertaken by racehorses. In addition, it is known that low forage rations lead to reduced bodyweights and corresponding improvements in performance due to reduced work efforts (Ellis *et al.*, 2002).

Further research is needed to identify whether there is an optimal forage: concentrate ratio that could minimise the detrimental effects of such diets on health and welfare, whilst maximizing the potential performance benefits observed in the present study.

In conclusion, forage:concentrate ratio has significant effects on racehorse acid-base metabolism and performance, with potential negative effects on the health and welfare of animals and enhancing effects on performance.

References

Baker, J.C., D.R. Topliff and D.W. Freeman, 1992. Effects of dietary cation-anion balance on acid-base balance and blood parameters in anaerobically exercised horses. Proc. Eq. Nutr. And Phys. Symp. 13: 191.

Cirelli, A.A., 1993. Principles of nutrition for the performance horse. Equine Athlete 6: 13-14.

Eaton, M.D., D.R. Hodgson, D.L. Evans, W,L. Bryden and R.J. Rose, 1995. Effect of a diet containing supplementary fat on the capacity for high intensity exercise. Equine Vet. J. Suppl. 18: 353-356.

Ellis, J.M., T. Hollands and D.E. Allen, 2002. Effect of forage intake on bodyweight and performance. Equine Vet. J. Suppl. 34: 66-70.

Garner, H.E., D.P. Hutcheson, J.R. Coffman, A.W. Hahn and C. Salem, 1977. Lactic acidosis: a factor associated with equine laminitis. J. Anim. Sci. 45: 1037-1041.

Glade, M.J., 1983. Nutrition and performance of racing thoroughbreds. Equine Vet. J. 15: 31-36.

Harris, P.A., 1999. Review of equine feeding and stable management practices in the UK concentrating on the last decade of the 20th century. Equine Vet. J. Suppl. 28: 46-54.

Graham-Thiers, P.M., D.S. Kronfeld and K.A. Kline, 1999. Dietary protein influences acid-base responses to repeated sprints. Equine Vet. J. Suppl. 30: 463-467.

Jackson, J.A., V. Akay, S.T. Franklin and D.K. Aaron, 2001. The effect of cation-anion difference on calcium requirement, feed intake, bodyweight gain, and blood gasses and mineral concentrations in dairy calves. J. Dairy Sci. 84: 147-153.

Kienzle, E., 1994. Small intestinal digestion of starch in the horse. Revue Med. Vet. 145: 199-204.

MacLeay, J.M., S.J. Valberg, J.D. Pagan, J.L. Xue, F.D. De La Corte and J. Roberts, 2000. Effect of ration and exercise on plasma creatine kinase activity and lactate concentration in Thoroughbred horses with recurrent exertional rhabdomyolysis. Am. J. vet. Res. 61: 1390-1395.

McLean, B.M.L., J.J. Hyslop, A.C. Longland and D. Cuddeford, 1998. Effects of physical processing of barley and its effects on intra-caecal pH and volatile fatty acid parameters in ponies offered barley-based diets. Proc. Of the 2nd Annual Conference of the European Society of Veterinary and Comparative Nutrition, 61.

Radicke, S., E. Landes, E. Kienzle and H. Meyer, 1992. Aktivitat der amylase im Darmkanal des Pferdes in Abhangigkeit des pferdes. Europasche Konferenz uber die Ernahrung des Pferdes 1: 99-102.

Tinker, M.K., NA. White, P. Lessard, C.D. Thatcher, K.D. Pelzer, B. Davis and D.K. Carmel, 1997. Prospective study of equine colic risk factors. Equine Vet. J. 29: 454-458.

Tucker, W.B., G.A. Harrison and R.W. Hemkin, 1988. Influence of dietary cation-anion balance on milk, blood, urine and rumen fluid in lactating dairy cattle. J. Dairy Sci. 71: 346-354.

Willard, J.G., J.C. Willard, S.A. Wolfram and J.P. Baker, 1997. Effect of diet on caecal pH and feeding behaviour of horses. J. Anim. Sci. 45: 87.

Zeyner, A., H. Kirbach and M. Furll, 2002. Effects of substituting starch with fat on the acid-base and mineral status of female horses. Equine Vet. J. Suppl. 34: 85-94.

Training and competition follow-up in the field in young horses trained for three-day-eventing

Anne Couroucé-Malblanc[1], Elsa Authié[1], Benjamin Morillon[1] and Sophie Biau[2]
[1]Ecole Nationale Vétérinaire de Nantes, Unité de nutrition et endocrinologie, Atlanpôle – La Chantrerie, 44307 Nantes cedex, France; courouce@vet-nantes.fr
[2]Ecole Nationale d'Equitation, Terrefort, St Hilaire St Florent, BP 207, 49400 Saumur, France

Take home message

In young horses trained for three-day-eventing, there is an important difference between workload during training and workload during competition.

Purpose of work

Three-day-eventing horses take part of important competitions when they are more than 7 years old. However, at 4 and 5 years old (yo), horses start daily training and take part in competitions designed for young horses. Very little is known about their training and competition. The aim of this study was to measure workload during training and competition in young horses trained for three-day-eventing.

Material and methods

A total of 13 young horses from the eventing stable of the National Equestrian School (Saumur) were followed from April to June in 2006 and 2007. In 2006, four 4-yo horses, in 2007 four 4-yo» and five 5-yo horses were monitored. Heart rate (HR) was measured throughout training and competition using a Polar heart rate meter (Polar S610, Polar, Finland). For some exercises, velocity was measured with a GPS device (Garmin). Also, blood samples were collected from the jugular vein to measure blood lactate concentration (Accutrend, Roche). For each horse, exercise duration, recovery duration, rider and groom impressions were written down in a training pad.

Results

The results showed great variability of the exercise. The aim of the rider, as well as HR, velocity and blood lactate concentration measurements helped to distinguish 12 types of exercises: dressage, endurance, cross, gallop, unrestricted work, lunge work, trotting, recovery, jumping (work over obstacles), jumping (gymnastics), walk. Also, competitions were followed: combination of dressage and jumping for 4-yo, cross country for 4 and 5-yo and also show jumping.

In 2006 mean heart was below 120 bpm for all exercises except for gallop for which mean HR (± SD) was 158 (± 26) bpm. Mean blood lactate concentration was lower than 1 mmol/l for all exercises except for gallop for which mean blood lactate concentration (± SD) was 3.0 (± 1.2) mmol/l. However, very few gallops were realised by young horses. For competition (cross country), mean HR (± SD) was 214 (± 11) bpm and mean blood lactate concentration (± SD) was 9.0 (± 3.5) mmol/l.

In 2007, 4- and 5-yo were considered as young horses and compared to mature horses (five 7-yo monitored). There was no effect of age on mean HR and also on HR intervals expressed as a percentage considering either all exercises and also according to the different exercises. Also, exercises were analysed according to HR values with the following HR intervals: HR < 90 bpm; 90 bpm < HR < 130 bpm; 130 bpm < HR < 160 bpm; HR > 160 bpm. These HR intervals were defined to evaluate different work intensities. For all horses and all exercises performed during training, 50% of the work was performed with a HR below 90 bpm; 37% with a HR between 90 and 130 bpm; 9.4% with a HR between 130 and 160 bpm and 3.6% with a HR over 160 bpm. The percentage of HR over 160 bpm for 4- and 5-yo was respectively 1.6% and 1.9%. For 7-yo, this percentage was higher: 7.7%. Also, duration of dressage and jumping (work over obstacles) was significantly lower for young horses compared to mature horses (P<0.05). The duration of gallops could not be compared between young and mature horses as very few gallops were performed by 4- and 5-yo.

Discussion

The results of this study show that there were few exercise sessions resulting in blood lactate concentrations between 2 and 4 mmol/l (Couroucé, 1998, 1999; Leleu *et al.*, 2005). This kind of work could be included in endurance or canter exercises. It could help to increase the horse's aerobic capacity and thus delay blood lactate accumulation (Couroucé, 1998). Also, results during competition show a much higher workload compared to training. This study shows an important difference between what is asked to the horse during training and during competition. Veterinary files show that, in 2007, there was an interruption of training in July for two of the four 4-yo (one due to orthopaedic and one due to respiratory problems) and also for four of the five 5-yo (three due to tendonitis and one due to gastric ulcers). Fatigue could be the cause of some of these diseases (Leleu *et al.*, 2005).

References

Couroucé, A., 1998. Endurance and sprint training. In Proceedings: Conference on Equine Sports Medicine and Science (CESMAS): 190-202.

Couroucé, A., 1999. Field Exercise testing for assessing fitness in French Standardbred trotters, The Veterinary Journal, 157: 112-122.

Leleu, C., C. Cotrel and A. Couroucé-Malblanc, 2005. Relationships between physiological variables and race performance in French standardbred trotters. The Veterinary Record, 156: 339-342.

Cortisol response of therapeutic riding horses to hippotherapy and horse riding sessions

C. Cravana, F. Di Giovanni, P. Medica, E. Fazio and A. Ferlazzo
Department of Morphology, Biochemistry, Physiology and Animal Production, Unit of Veterinary Physiology, Faculty of Veterinary Medicine, University of Messina, Italy

Take home message

Cortisol concentrations may be used as stress marker during hippotherapy sessions. In trained therapeutic riding horses the cortisol levels during hippotherapy session were lower than during horse riding sessions.

Introduction

Hippotherapy is an animal-assisted therapy supporting or reinforcing motor, biochemical, cognitive, emotional and social functions in disabled people. It is considered as a direct medical treatment (NARHA, 2002).

Hippotherapy provides many benefits for the patient, such as improvements to posture, balance and sensorimotor programming (Benda *et al.*, 2003; Meregillano, 2004). Additional benefits are motivation, bonding and communication between horse and rider (Debuse *et al.*, 2005).

In spite of the large utilization of this kind of therapy in human medicine, little scientific research has been made about the potential detrimental effects caused to the horses utilized in the course of therapeutic activities (Anderson *et al.*, 1999; Casciana *et al.*, 2005; Kaiser *et al.*, 2006).

In horses, glucocorticoides are important physiological variables commonly used for the evaluation of stress response (Foreman and Ferlazzo, 1996; De Vries *et al.*, 2000; Hada *et al.*, 2003). Physical exercise is known to induce an increase in circulating cortisol levels (Ferlazzo and Fazio, 1997; Ferlazzo *et al.*, 2007). Moreover, adrenocortical response is greatly involved in psychological stress in competitive events (Ferlazzo *et al.*, 1998; Fazio *et al.*, 2000), as well as during transportation (Friend *et al.*,1998; Cusumano *et al.*, 2001) and during confinement and isolation (Fazio *et al.*, 2001; Cusumano *et al.*, 2004).

The aim of this study was to investigate whether trained therapeutic riding horses (TRH) showed different patterns of cortisol changes during two different treatments represented by hippotherapy and horse riding sessions.

Materials and methods

Three healthy Sella Italiana female horses, aged 18 years, weighing 475±23 (SD) kg were studied. All horses were trained both for therapy and horse riding activity since 6 years. During three weeks, all horses were submitted to two different treatments, hippotherapy sessions (Session A) and horse riding sessions for beginners (Session B). Each session lasted 15 minutes. Session A consisted of different actions like walk, trotting, halting and individualized therapy activities with the therapist. During the Session B every horse was submitted to exercise consisting of 5 min walk, 5 min trotting and 5 min galloping. Both sessions were carried out inside an enclosed arena (32.77 m wide x 71.33 m long) and all doors leading into the arena were closed. During the session A the riders were paediatric patients affected by various cognitive and sensory disabilities (psychoneurosis, depression, psychosis). During the Session B the riders were healthy children. The sessions were conducted by two licensed therapists and one professional horseman. In order to evaluate the individual response, the two treatments were repeated on each horse once a week for three consecutive weeks. During each week, all TRH horses were submitted to Session A and after 3 days to session B.

Blood samples were collected from jugular vein by indwelling catheter, prior to the session, at 09.00 a.m., in basal conditions, and at the mounting, at 5 min,10 min and 15 min during the activity, at the end of the session in the box and 5 min and 30 min after the session. Serum cortisol concentrations were analysed in duplicate by immunoenzymatic assay (RADIM).

During the sessions, the heart rate was measured by Polar Equine Heart Rate Monitor S-610 (Polar Electro Europe BV). Heart rate was recorded every three minutes.

Statistics: to determine the effect of the treatments over time, an analysis of variance for repeated measures (RM ANOVA) was applied. To compare post-session to basal values the paired t-test was applied. The level of significance was set at <0.05.

Results

The patterns of mean cortisol levels of TRH horses during Session A (hippotherapy sessions) and Session B (horse riding sessions) are shown in Figure 1.

In session A mean serum cortisol concentrations were significant lower than in session B in basal conditions, at mounting, at 5 min ($p<0.01$) and at 10 min ($p<0.02$) during the activity and 5 min and 30 min ($p<0.02$) after the activity.

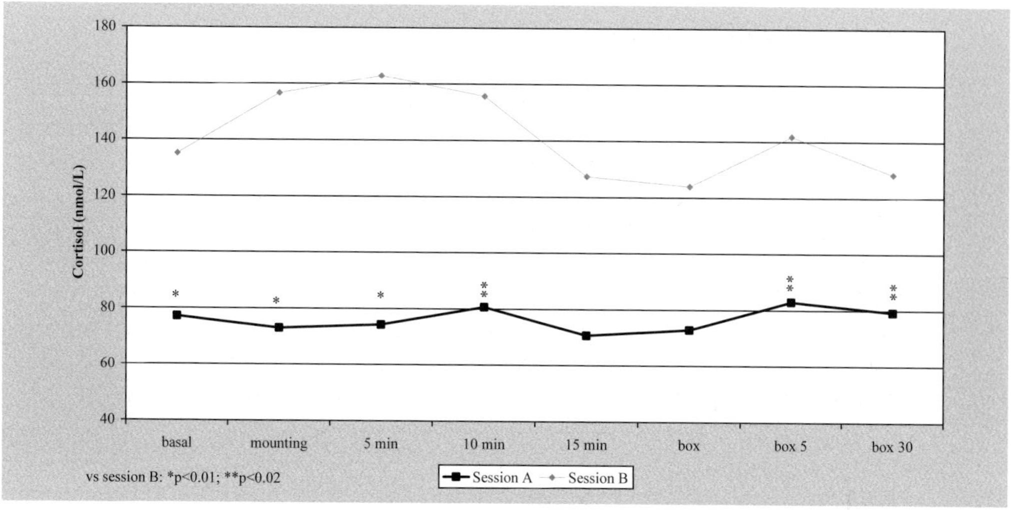

Figure 1. Mean serum cortisol levels of Therapeutic Riding Horses (TRH) in session A (hippotherapy sessions) and session B (horse riding sessions) during three consecutive weeks.

In session A, compared to basal values, mean cortisol levels showed increases at 10 min during the therapeutic activity, and 5 min and 30 min after the session, and decreases at mounting, at 5 min, at 15 min during the activity, and at the return in the box. No significant differences between the different times were found.

In Session B, compared to basal values, mean cortisol levels showed an increase at mounting, at 5 min and at 10 min during the activity and 5 min after the session, and decreases at 15 min during the activity, at the return in the box and 30 min after the session. No significant differences between the different times were found.

RM-ANOVA showed significant effects in both Session A ($F=36.88$; $p<0.0001$) and Session B ($F=28.24$; $p<0.0001$) on mean circulating cortisol changes.

The patterns of mean heart rate values of TRH horses during Session A and Session B are shown in Figure 2.

In session A the mean heart rate values at 10 min and at 15 min during the activity were significantly lower than in session B ($p<0.01$).

In both sessions, compared to basal values, mean heart rate values showed increases at all sampling times during and after the activity. No significant differences between the different times were found.

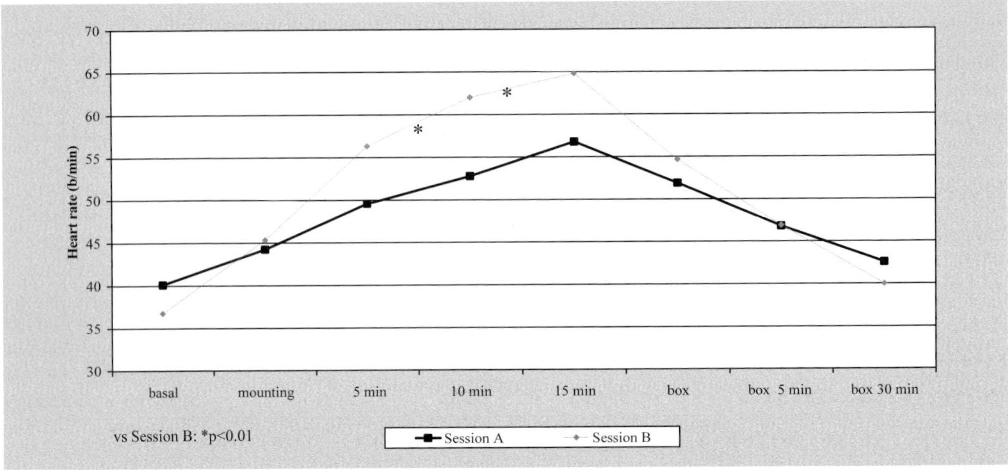

Figure 2. Mean heart rate values of Therapeutic Riding Horse (TRH) in session A (hippotherapy sessions) and session B (horse riding sessions) during three consecutive weeks.

In session A heart rate averaged between 39 and 57 beats per minute and in session B it averaged between 37 and 65 beats per minute.

RM-ANOVA showed significant effects in both Session A (F=25.02; p<0.0001) and Session B (F=35.90; p<0.0001) on mean heart rate.

The evaluation of the cortisol changes in each horse in the 3 weeks of study showed that the pattern was similar during the hippotherapy sessions, while it varied a lot during the horse riding sessions. On the contrary, a similar pattern of individual heart rate changes was observed during both sessions in the 3 weeks of study.

Discussion

The basal cortisol levels were significantly lower before hippotherapy than before horse riding session. This may reflect the individual coping capacity for stress of horses. Also the cortisol levels were lower during hippotherapy than during horse riding sessions. This may have been due to the different role of the riders in controlling the direction and cadence of horses. Possibly the activity with children suffering from cognitive and sensory disabilities represents a minor stress in TRH horses than the activity with able bodied children.

These data are in agreement with previous data obtained in TRH horses (Casciana *et al.*, 2005), showing higher cortisol levels during hippotherapy sessions for patients suffering from motor disabilities than during hippotherapy sessions for patients suffering from cognitive and sensory disabilities.

During horse riding sessions the mean cortisol levels were higher than during hippotherapy reflecting the higher intensity of physical activity requested during horse riding sessions (Ferlazzo and Fazio, 1997; Fazio *et al.*, 1999; Lindner *et al.*, 2002), as well as in Thoroughbreds during and after SET on a treadmill (Lindner *et al.*, 2000; Medica *et al.*, 2002).

The cortisol levels increased faster during horse riding sessions than hippotherapy sessions. In fact, the TRH horses showed high emotional involvement during horse riding session, like sport horses prior and during competition. These data confirm data observed as an effect of psychological stress in show jumping horses (Aronica *et al.*, 1999) and in Thoroughbreds and Standardbreds (Cravana *et al.*, 2006, 2007) prior and after competitive events.

All TRH horses showed higher heart rates during horse riding sessions as compared to hippotherapy sessions. These may again reflect the different typology of riders.

It should be noted that overall the heart rate increases were relatively moderate and well within aerobic ranges during both sessions. The activities carried out during both sessions did not represent high degrees of stress condition in TRH horses.

Further evaluation needs the possibility of distinguishing between psychic and physical stress by measuring concurrently the serum cortisol concentration and heart rate.

References

Anderson, M.K., T.H. Friend, J.W. Evans and D.M. Bushong, 1999. Appl Anim Behav Sci; 63: 11-24.

Aronica, V., E. Fazio, R. Di Majo, L. Grasso and A. Ferlazzo, 1999. Atti SO.F.I.VET 3: 65-69.

Benda, W., N.H. Mc Gibbon and K.L. Grant, 2003. J Alternative and Complementary Med. 9: 817-25.

Casciana, L., E. Fazio, P. Medica, C. Cravana and A. Ferlazzo, 2005. Atti Accad. Pelor. Peric., XCIII: 47-55.

Cravana, C., P. Medica, E. Fazio, F. Di Giovanni and A. Ferlazzo, 2006. In: A. Lindner (Ed.) Management of lameness causes in sport horses, Wageningen Academic Publishers, the Netherlands, p. 165-168.

Cravana, C., E. Fazio, P. Medica, A. Sofia and A. Ferlazzo, 2007. Att. Soc. it. Sci. vet., 93-94.

Cusumano, F., E. Fazio and A. Ferlazzo, 2001. Proc 6th Annual Congress of the European College of Sport Science, 902.

Cusumano, F., E. Fazio, P. Medica, L. Grasso and A. Ferlazzo, 2004. Proc. 54th Annual Meeting of the Eur. Assoc. for Animal Production, 9: 396.

Debuse, D., C. Chandler and C. Gibb, 2005. Physiotherapy, Theory and Practice, 21: 219-42.

De Vries, W.R., N.T. Bernards, M.H. de Rooij and H.P. Koppeschaar, 2000. Psychosom Med 62: 866-872.

Fazio, E., P. Medica, A. Lindner and A. Ferlazzo, 1999. Atti SO.F.I.VET 3: 55-59.

Fazio, E., D. Alberghina, V. Aronica, P. Medica and A. Ferlazzo, 2000. In: A. Lindner (Ed.) The elite show jumper, Wageningen Academic Publishers, the Netherlands, p. 113-115.

Fazio, E., L. Grasso, D. Alberghina and A. Ferlazzo, 2001. SISVet Annual Meeting Selected Abstracts, III: 56-57.

Ferlazzo, A. and E. Fazio, 1997. In: A. Lindner (Ed.) Performance diagnosis of horses. Wageningen Pers, Wageningen, the Netherlands, p. 30-43.

Ferlazzo, A., E. Fazio, V. Aronica, R. Di Majo, P. Medica and I. Grasso, 1998. In: A. Lindner (Ed.) Proc. 2nd Conf. on Equine Sports Medicine and Science, 53-56.

Ferlazzo, A., P. Medica and E. Fazio, 2007. In: F. Boffi (Ed.) Fisiologia del Ejercicio en Equinos. Parte II. Cap. 11, Editorial Inter-Médica S.A.I.C.I., Buenos Aires, República Argentina, p. 153-164.

Foreman, J.H. and A. Ferlazzo, 1996. Pferdeheilkunde, 12: 401-404.

Friend, T.H., M.T. Martin, D.D. Householder and D.M. Bushong, 1998. J Am Vet Med Assoc, 212: 838-44.

Hada, T., T. Onaka, T. Takahashi, A. Hiraga and K. Yagi, 2003. J Neuroendocrinol 15: 638-648.

Kaiser, L., C.R. Heleski, J. Siegford and K.A. Smith, 2006. J Am Vet Med Assoc, 228: 39-45.

Lindner, A., E. Fazio, A.M. Ferlazzo, P. Medica and A. Ferlazzo, 2000. Pferdeilkunde 16: 502-510.

Lindner, A., E. Fazio, P. Medica and A. Ferlazzo, 2002. Pferdeheilkunde 18: 51-56.

Medica, P., D. Alberghina, E. Fazio, S.J. Wickler and A. Ferlazzo, 2002. Atti Soc it Sci vet 56: 83-84.

Meregillano, G., 2004. Hippotherapy. Phys Med Rehabil Clin N Am; 15:843-54.

NARHA, 2002. NARHA Instructor Educational Guide. North American Riding for the Handicapped Association, Inc., eds. Denver (CO).

The influences of overtraining on the hypothalamo-pituitary-adrenocortical axis in Standardbred horses

E. de Graaf-Roelfsema[1], H.A. Keizer[2], E. van Breda[3], I.D. Wijnberg[1] and J.H. van der Kolk[1]
[1]Department of Equine Sciences, Medicine Section, Faculty of Veterinary Medicine, Utrecht University, The Netherlands
[2]Department of Human Physiology and Sportsmedicine, Free University of Brussels, Brussel, Belgium
[3]Department of Human Movement Sciences, Faculty of Health, Medicine and Life Sciences, Maastricht University, The Netherlands

Take home message

Overtraining leads to a dysfunction of the HPA axis in Standardbred horses possibly related to increased secretion of CRH.

Introduction

Alterations in functioning of the HPA axis has been described in trained, overreached and overtrained horses. Several mechanisms underlying the alterations in functioning have been suggested, among them diminished adrenocortical sensitivity to ACTH and decreased negative feedback sensitivity. However, so far only ACTH challenges were used to study the alterations in the HPA axis in horses during training and in order to define the location and nature of the alteration(s) a more central stimulator of the HPA axis like corticotropin releasing hormone (CRH) seems to be needed. The current study investigated the influences of overtraining on the function of the HPA axis using a CRH-stimulation test in Standardbred horses.

Material and methods

A longitudinal training study with ten 1.5 year old Standardbred geldings was performed on a treadmill for a total of 32 weeks. Training was divided into four periods:

- acclimatisation;
- training;
- intensified training;
- detraining.

In period 3, the horses were randomly divided into 2 groups: control (C) and intensified trained (IT) group. At the end of period 1 and period 3 Corticotropin

Releasing Factor (CRF, C-3042, Sigma-Aldrich Chemie BV, Zwijndrecht, The Netherlands) 0.01 μg/kg BW was administered intravenously. Blood was sampled before administration of CRF, and 5, 10 and 300 minutes post-injection for determination of plasma ACTH and/or cortisol concentrations. The overtraining status was evaluated by means of a standardized exercise and behavioral tests.

Plasma cortisol and ACTH concentrations were measured by use of a radioimmunoassay validated for use in samples obtained from horses.

Statistical analysis was performed using a linear mixed-effects model with a one-step autoregressive process. Fixed factors used were horse, couple, group and period. P value < 0.05 was considered significant.

Results

The ACTH concentration at 10 minutes after CRF administration corrected for the pre-injection concentration was significantly lower for the overtrained horses compared to the control group after period 3 (Table 1). Plasma cortisol concentrations (corrected as well as not corrected) did not show significant differences for group or period.

The diagnosis of overtraining was based on a significant reduction in total trot time (19%) during a standardised treadmill exercise test for the intensified trained horses. The condition was distinguished from short-term fatigue or overreaching

Table 1. Results of hCRH stimulation test in a control group (C) and an intensified trained (IT) group measured at rest after acclimatization phase (1) and a training period of 24 weeks (C3) or training period of 18 weeks directly followed by an intensified training period of 6 weeks (IT 3). All data are corrected for pre-injection concentrations and presented as mean ± sd.

	Group/phase	0 min	5 min	10 min
Δ Plasma ACTH	C 1	0	41 ± 20	32 ± 45
	IT 1	0	74 ± 64	65 ± 36
	C 3	0	73 ± 67	88 ± 63[a]
	IT 3	0	31 ± 12.5	38 ± 12[b]
Δ Plasma cortisol	C 1	0	31 ± 14	117 ± 98
	IT 1	0	29 ± 33	65 ± 50
	C 3	0	17 ± 23	107 ± 44
	IT 3	0	-1.2 ± 35	60 ± 67

[ab] means values significant different (P<0.05).

by the demonstration of a persistent reduction in performance capacity after 4 weeks of detraining. Overtraining was also associated with behavioural changes of internal conflict in the overtrained horses indicating mental stress.

Conclusions

The main finding was a reduction in the ACTH response to administration of CRH in the overtrained group. This finding was not accompanied by significant differences between the control and IT group in plasma cortisol concentrations after CRF administration. The results confirm the hypothesis that overtraining in Standardbred horses is associated with dysfunction of the HPA axis. Since the corrected plasma cortisol levels after administration of CRF were the same for the control and the OT group and the corrected ACTH levels were significantly lower for the overtrained horses, the OT horses seem to have a relatively higher cortisol response to the ACTH released during CRH stimulation. This correlates with findings in patients with anorexia nervosa and other stress-related disorders. Since basal concentrations of ACTH and cortisol were normal, negative feedback mechanism of cortisol on the pituitary gland functioned. Therefore, the decrease in pituitary sensitivity must be caused by a more centrally located disorder like directly by long-term increased CRH secretion raised by chronic stress or indirectly by increased secretion of an ACTH inhibitory factor that counteracts the action of CRH raised by chronic social stress as described by Alexander *et al.* (1996) in chronic socially stressed horses.

References

Alexander, S.L., C.H.G. Irvine and R.A. Donald, 1996. Dynamics of the regulation of the Hypothalamo-pituitary-adrenal (HPA) axis determined using a nonsurgical method for collecting pituitary venous blood from horses. Frontiers in neuroendocrinology 17: 1-50.

The effect of overtraining and subsequent detraining on glucose metabolism and peripheral insulin sensitivity in Standardbred horses

E. de Graaf-Roelfsema[1], H.A. Keizer[2], E. van Breda[3], I.D. Wijnberg[1] and J.H. van der Kolk[1]
[1]Department of Equine Sciences, Medicine Section, Faculty of Veterinary Medicine, Utrecht University, Yalelaan 114, 3508 TD Utrecht, the Netherlands
[2]Department of Human Physiology and Sportsmedicine, Free University of Brussels, Brussel, Belgium
[3]Department of Movement Sciences, Faculty of Health Sciences, University of Maastricht, the Netherlands

Take home message

The demonstration of dissociation between glucose metabolism and insulin sensitivity in individual subjects might indicate overtraining.

Introduction

Insulin sensitivity indirectly correlates with glucose metabolism via glucose transporter 4. Physical training has been associated with alterations in glucose tolerance and insulin action. The aim of the current study was to assess glucose metabolism and peripheral insulin sensitivity in experimentally induced overtraining in Standardbreds according to a previously described protocol characterised by insufficient rest days.

Material and methods

A longitudinal training study with ten Standardbred geldings (20 ± 2sd months old) was performed on a high-speed treadmill for a total of 32 weeks. Training was divided into four periods:

- acclimatisation;
- training;
- intensified training;
- detraining.

Horses were randomly assigned to either the intensified training program or served as a matched control by continuing current training.

At the end of each period, both a standardised exercise test (SET) and an euglycaemic hyperinsulinaemic clamp test were performed in each horse. Statistical analysis was done using a linear mixed-effects model and the Pearson product moment correlation test (2-tailed). P values < 0.05 were considered significant.

Results

Intensified trained horses showed a 19% decrease ($P = 0.012$) in performance during SET3 associated with dissociation between glucose metabolism and insulin sensitivity ($r = 0.812$ and $P = 0.095$ compared with $r = 0.987$ and $P = 0.002$ in controls) and this dissociation persisted after four weeks of detraining.

Conclusion

Overtraining in Standardbred horses was associated with dissociation between glucose metabolism and insulin sensitivity persisting after four weeks of detraining.

Circulating cortisol levels of Arab sport horses before and after gymkana riding events: effects of training state, gender and age

E. Fazio, P. Molinari, P. Medica, C. Messineo and A. Ferlazzo
Department of Morphology, Biochemistry, Physiology and Animal Production, Unit of Physiology, Faculty of Veterinary Medicine, University of Messina, Italy

Take home message

Cortisol concentrations may provide additional information for the monitoring of gymkana riding performance.

Introduction

Gymkana exercise is one the most popular equestrian events in which sport horses are currently utilized. The type of western show activities and of performance horses can be categorized in many different ways. The spectrum of western show horses is represented by Cutting and Reining Horses, Team Roping and Steer Wrestling Horses, Barrel Racing and Gymkana Horses, Western Pleasure and Trail Show Horses. There are significant differences in horse conformation and body type depending upon the performance discipline.

Gymkana requires speed and agility over a short course. Typical conformation is of the 'sprint horse' type, with many of these horses deriving from Arabian Breed. These physical activities are represented by both anaerobic and aerobic work, requiring maximal muscular contractions and motor ability for a very short time.

It is well known that cortisol is considered a marker of psycho-physical stress in horses (Foreman and Ferlazzo, 1996) and that exercise induces significant modifications of cortisol levels (Ferlazzo and Fazio, 1997; Ferlazzo *et al.*, 2007). Cortisol levels are also considered physiological markers for evaluating training status in warmblood horses (Marc *et al.*, 2000) and for performance diagnosis in Thoroughbred horses during and after standardized exercise tests (SET) on treadmill (Lindner *et al.*, 2000).

On this basis, the purpose of this study was to evaluate the effects of gymkana competition on circulating cortisol concentrations in trained and untrained Arabian breed horses, by taking into account the effects of gender and age.

Materials and methods

A total of twenty-three healthy Arabian breed horses (9 trained and 14 untrained horses) of different gender (12 females and 11 males) and age (thirteen 4-9 years old and ten 10-15 years old) were submitted to conventional training for gymkana riding.

Trained horses were submitted to an exercise protocol once a week for 4 weeks. After a warm-up of 5 min walking, the exercise protocol was represented by:

- 1st week= Conventional exercise on the track for 90 min (30 min walk, 20 min trot, 10 min canter and 30 min walk).
- 2nd week= Conventional exercise on the track for 45 min (15 min walk, 10 min trot, 5 min gallop, 15 min trot and gallop on the track).
- 3rd week= Simulated Gimkana competition for 10 min on the race track.
- 4th week= Final exercise for 90 min, before the competition (30 min walk, 20 min trot, 5 min canter, 5 min free gallop, 30 min walk).

The challenge or difficulty of a category varied according to the number of exercise steps into gymkana race track (Figure 1) and riders were advised to know the general difficulty of a trail before starting the ride.

Trained horses belonged to *Pro* (14 exercises) and *Semipro* (11 exercises, except exercise in 4, 5 and 10 steps) categories, on the basis of the different number of exercises and of the ability of riders; untrained horses belonged only to *Junior* (9 exercises, except exercise in 1, 4, 5, 10, 13 steps) category, on the basis of the age of rider (*Under 16*).

Untrained horses were submitted to training for 1 week just before the gymkana competition: 5 min warm-up, 10 min walk, 10 min trot, 5 min gallop and 15 min trot and gallop.

Blood samples were collected from jugular vein prior to the gymkana competition, at 09.00 a.m., in basal conditions, and 5 and 30 min after the competition. Serum cortisol concentrations were analysed in duplicate by immunoenzymatic assay (RADIM).

Statistics: data are presented as mean ± standard deviation (SD). To compare basal values with post-exercise values, an analysis of variance for repeated measures (RM-ANOVA) was applied. To determine the effects of gymkana competition on training status, gender and age an one way analysis of variance (ANOVA) was applied. The level of significance was set at <0.05. The percentage differences (Δ%) were also calculated.

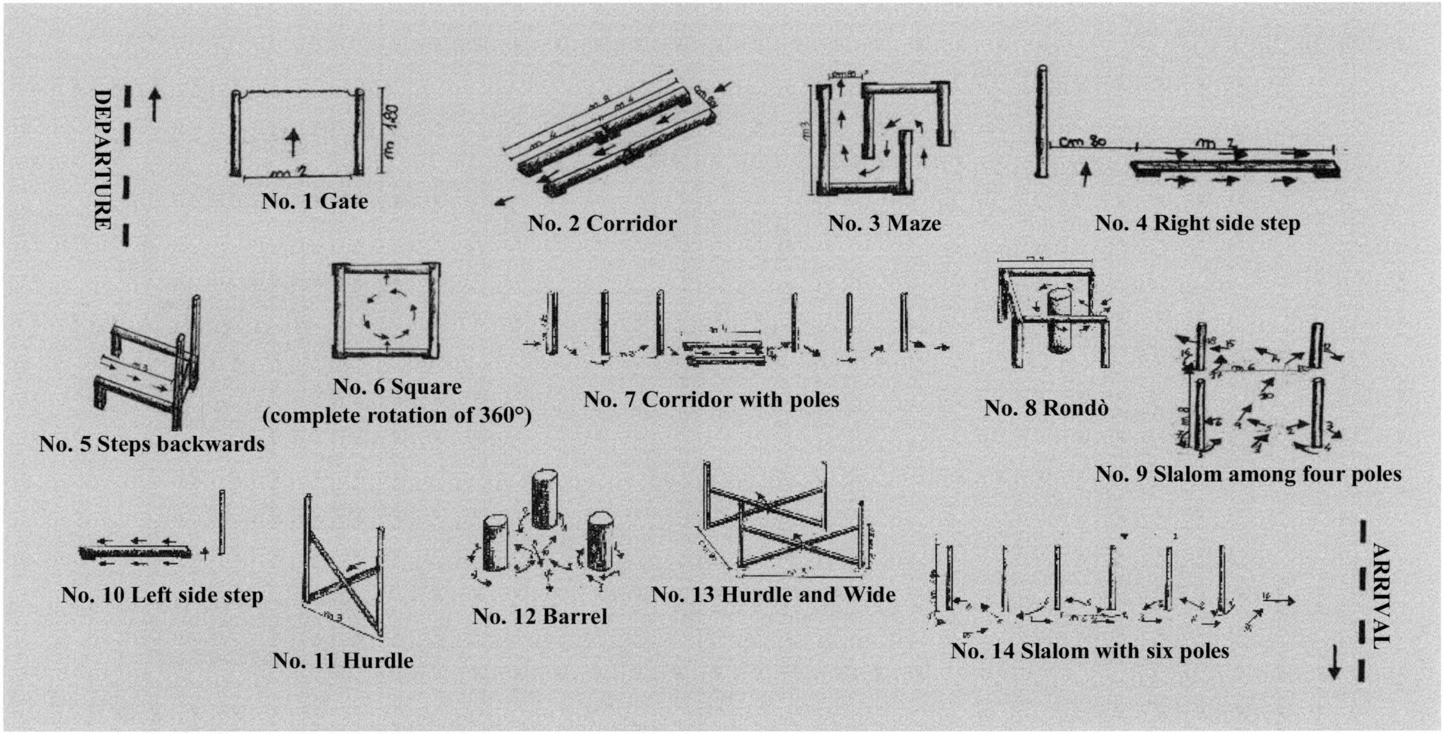

Figure 1. The race course of gimkana riding events.

Results

The effects of gymkana exercise on mean cortisol levels in trained and untrained horses are shown in Figure 2. Compared to basal values, an increase of serum cortisol concentration was observed in the trained horses 5 min (+27.00%) and 30 min (+72.44%; $p<0.001$) after exercise and in the untrained horses 5 min (+30.46%; $p<0.05$) and 30 min (+43.91%; $p<0.01$) after exercise. ANOVA for repeated measures showed a significant effect of exercise on cortisol changes both in trained ($F=14.38$; $p<0.001$) and untrained ($F=22.57$; $p<0.001$) horses. However, there were no significant differences between trained and untrained horses.

The patterns of cortisol levels in female and male horses are shown in Figure 3. In mares serum cortisol concentration increased 5 min (+30.46%) and 30 min (+38.08%; <0.001) after exercise, and in males 5 min (+28.01%) and 30 min (+90.80%; $p<0.01$) after exercise. ANOVA for repeated measures showed significant effects of exercise on cortisol changes both in females ($F=11.49$; $p<0.001$) and males ($F=34.62$; $p<0.001$). In addition, males showed higher cortisol levels than mares 30 min after exercise ($P<0.05$).

The effect of age is shown in Figure 4. Serum cortisol concentration increased in horses aged 4-9 years 5 min (+25.86%) and 30 min (+72.10%; <0.001) after exercise, and in horses aged 10-15 years 5 min (+33.83%) and 30 min (+81.85%; $p<0.01$) after exercise. ANOVA for repeated measures showed a significant effect of exercise on cortisol changes in both age groups, but there were no significant differences between the age groups.

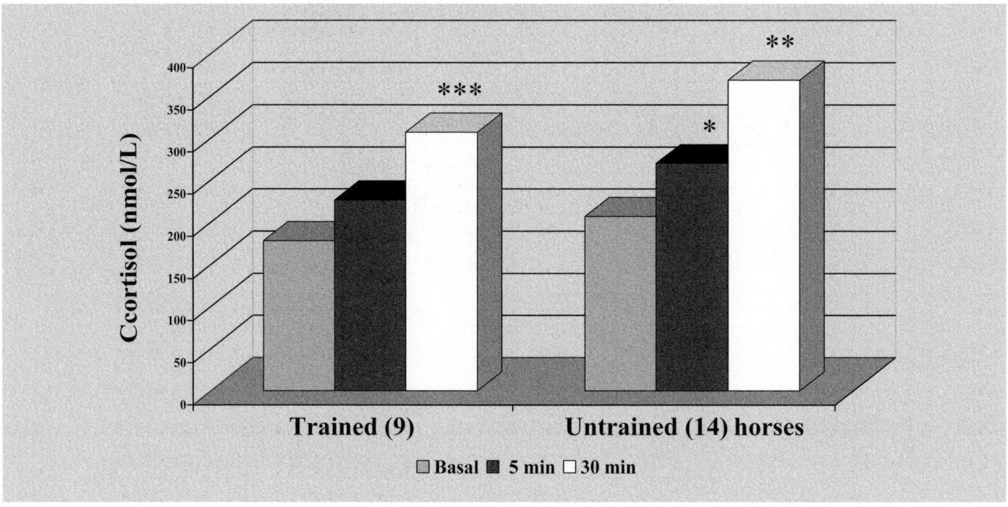

Figure 2. Serum cortisol levels before and after gimkana competition in trained and untrained Arab horses.

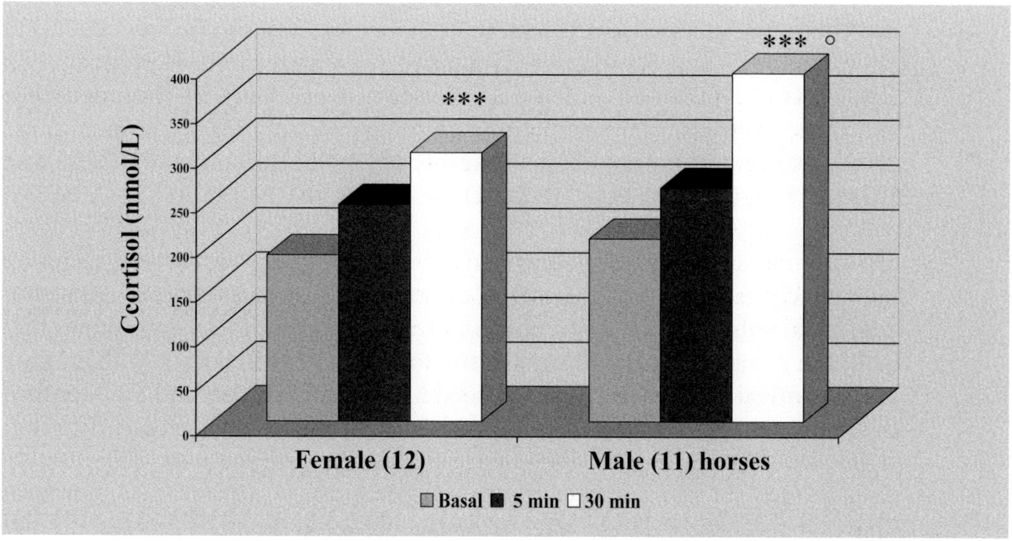

Figure 3. Serum cortisol levels before and after gimkana competition in female and male Arab horses.

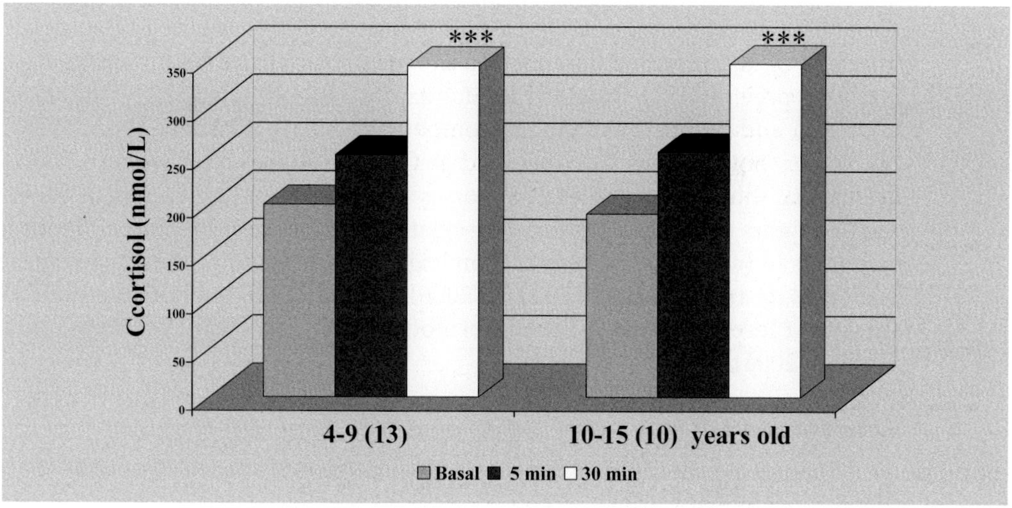

Figure 4. Serum cortisol levels before and after gimkana competition in Arab horses of different ages.

Discussion

The results obtained confirm the significant effect of exercise generally reported on circulating cortisol levels of sport horses (Ferlazzo and Fazio, 1997; Linden *et al.*, 1991; Nagata *et al.*, 1999; Green *et al.*, 2002; Medica *et al.*, 2004; Ferlazzo *et al.*, 2007). Increases of cortisol levels have been observed in jumpers after show jumping competition (Ferlazzo *et al.*, 1998; Fazio *et al.*, 2000; 2002), in Thoroughbreds and Standardbreds after SET on a treadmill (Lindner, 1992; Lindner *et al.*, 2000) and on the track (Lindner *et al.*, 2002), in Thoroughbreds and Standardbreds after competition (Desmecht *et al.*, 1996; Cravana *et al.*, 2006, 2007), after endurance (Lassourd *et al.*, 1996; Robson *et al.*, 2003) and after trekking (Alberghina *et al.*, 2001).

The training state has been shown to have an effect on the cortisol secretion rates which were higher than basal values at 30 min in trained horses and higher than basal values at 5 and 30 min in untrained horses. These data shows that gymkana competition was more stressful for the untrained horses, with an early adrenocortical response already recorded 5 min after exercise, and they confirm that training state induces different trends of cortisol level after exercise (Church *et al.*, 1987; Golland *et al.*, 1996; Medica *et al.*, 2004; Cravana *et al.*, 2006; 2007).

The higher cortisol levels after exercise observed in male horses do not confirm previous data that reported higher cortisol values in female than male Standardbreds after both final training and competition (Cravana *et al.*, 2007), and in females than geldings after exercise (Cartmill *et al.*, 2003).

The lack of significant differences observed among the different age groups confirms previous data obtained in Standardbreds both after SET (Lindner *et al.*, 2002) and competitive and no competitive events (Cravana *et al.*, 2006), but it does not confirm data obtained in Quarter Horses after western riding events, that showed cortisol levels in horses aged 7-20 years higher than in horses aged 3-6 years (Fazio *et al.*, 2006). Age-related modifications in neuroendocrine responses add an additional layer of complexity in understanding the physiological responses to stress (Malinowski *et al.*, 2006). Indeed, the oldest horses produced the lowest levels of stress-induced hormones, such as cortisol (McKeever and Gordon, 2004).

References

Alberghina, D., P. Medica and E. Fazio, 2001. Book of Abstracts of the 6thAnnual Congress of the European College of Sport Science, 15, p.902, Sport und Buch Strauss GmbH, Cologne, (Germany).

Cartmill, J.A., D.L. Thompson, W.A. Storer, L.R. Gentry and N.K. Huff, 2003. J. Anim. Sci., 81: 2311-2321.

Church, D.B., D.L. Evans, D.R. Lewis and R.J. Rose, 1987. In: J.R. Gillespie and N.E. Robinson (Eds.) Equine Exercise Physiology 2, ICEEP Publ., Davis, California, p. 506-515.

Cravana, C., P. Medica, E. Fazio, F. Di Giovanni and A. Ferlazzo, 2006. In: A. Lindner (Ed.) Management of lameness causes in sport horses, Wageningen Academic Publishers, Wageningen, the Netherlands, p. 165-168.

Cravana, C., E. Fazio, P. Medica, A. Sofia and A. Ferlazzo, 2007. Atti Soc. it. Sci. vet., 93-94.
Desmecht, D., A. Linden, H. Amory, T. Art and P. Lekeux, 1996. Vet. Res. Commun., 20: 371-379.
Fazio, E., D. Alberghina, V. Aronica, P. Medica and A. Ferlazzo, 2000. In: A. Lindner (Ed.) The Elite Show Jumper, pp. 113-115.
Fazio, E., P. Medica, V. Aronica, F. Cusumano and A. Ferlazzo, 2002. In: A. Lindner (Ed.) The Elite Dressage and Three-Day-Event Horse, pp. 123-127.
Fazio, E., G. Calabrò, P. Medica, C. Messineo and A. Ferlazzo, 2006. In: A. Lindner (Ed.) Management of lameness causes in sport horses, Wageningen Academic Publishers, Wageningen, the Netherlands, p. 175-179.
Ferlazzo, A. and E. Fazio, 1997. In: Arno Lindner (Ed.) Performance diagnosis of horses, Wageningen Pers, Wageningen, the Netherlands, p. 30-43.
Ferlazzo, A., E. Fazio, V. Aronica, R. Di Majo, P. Medica and L. Grasso, 1998. A. Lindner (Ed.) Proc. 2nd Conf. on Equine Sports Medicine and Science, p.53-56.
Ferlazzo, A., P. Medica and E. Fazio, 2007. In: F. Boffi (Ed.) Training del Caballo de desporte. Respuesta y Adaptación, Parte II. Cap.11, Editorial Intermedica Saici, p. 153-164.
Foreman, J.H. and A. Ferlazzo,1996. Pferdeheilkunde, 12: 401-404.
Golland, L.C., D.L. Evans, G.M. Stone, C.M. Tyler, R.J. Rose and D.R. Hodgson, 1996. Pferdeheilkunde, 12: 531-533.
Green, H.M., E.A. Cogger, T.L. Miltenberger, A.K. Koch, R.E. Bray and S.J. Wickler, 2002. Equine vet. J., Suppl., 545-550.
Lassourd, V., V. Gayrard, V. Laroute, M. Alvinerie, P. Benard, D. Courtot and P.L. Toutain, 1996. Am. J. Physiol. Regul. Integr. Comp. Physiol., 271: R25-R33.
Linden, A., T. Art, H. Amory, D. Desmecht and P. Lekeux,1991. In: S.G.B. Persson, A. Lindholm and L.B. Jeffcott (Eds.) Equine Exercise Physiology 3, ICEEP Publications, Uppsala, Sweden, p. 391-396.
Lindner, A., 1992. In: A. Ubaldi (Ed.) State of art in animal clinical Biochemistry, 5thCongress of Internat. Soc. Anim. Clin. Biochem., p. 327-332.
Lindner, A., E. Fazio, A.M. Ferlazzo, P. Medica and A. Ferlazzo, 2000. Pferdeheilkunde, 16: 502-510.
Lindner, A., E. Fazio, P. Medica and A. Ferlazzo, 2002. Pferdeheilkunde, 18: 51-56.
Malinowski, K., E.J. Shock, P. Rochelle, C.F. Kearns, P.D. Guirnalda and K.H. McKeever, 2006. Equine vet. J. Suppl., 36: 267-273.
Marc, M., N. Parvizi, F. Ellendorff, E. Kallweit and F. Elsaesser, 2000. J. Anim. Sci., 78: 1936-1946.
McKeever, K.H. and M.E. Gordon, 2004. In: K.W. Hinchcliff, A. Kaneps and R. Geor (Eds.) Equine Sports Medicine and Surgery: Basic and Clinical Sciences of the Equine Athlete, Elsevier, Philadelphia, p. 793-814.
Medica, P., C. Cravana, D. Alberghina, E. Fazio and A. Ferlazzo, 2004. In: A. Lindner (Ed.) The Elite Race and Endurance Horse, p. 196-200.
Nagata, S., F. Takeda, M. Kurosawa, K. Mima, A. Hiraga, M. Kai and K. Taya,1999. Equine vet. J. Suppl., 30: 570-574.
Robson, P.J., T.D. Alston and K.H. Myburgh, 2003. Equine vet. J., 35: 133-137.

Quantification of negative mental status of a horse during physical activity

F. Jansen, J. Van der Krogt, K. Van Loon, S. Quanten, D. Berckmans, M. Guarino and V. Avezzù
Division Monitor, Model & Manage Bioresponses (M3-BIORES), K.U. Leuven, Belgium

Introduction

In equine sports developing training methods to optimise the performance of horses is a very challenging process. Despite the fact that the physiological condition of horses can be measured quite accurately under laboratory conditions (e.g. VO_2 test,…), it is expected that the performance of horses is influenced by its mental status.

The objective of this research was to quantify a negative mental status, in this case fear, of a horse during training activity in a continuous and non-invasive way, based on the measurement of heart rate and physical activity.

Material and methods

The experiment carried out was made up of 5 blocks, each lasting for 5 minutes, where the gait of the horse varied as follows: walking-trotting-walking-trotting-walking. When walking, the horse was moving at an average speed of 5 km/h (1.39 m/s). When trotting, the horse's speed was augmented to an average of 10 km/h (2.78 m/s). During the second trotting part stress was applied to the horse by suddenly opening an umbrella, as used by other authors.

During the experiment the horse's heart rate and physical activity were continuously measured using the Polar Equine RS800, which measures heart rate (RR intervals), and the ActiGraph GT1M, which quantifies physical activity.

The relationship between the horse's physical activity and its heart rate was described by a single input – single output (SISO) mathematical model. The horse's physical activity was used as the input and its heart rate as the output. Since a horse can be considered as a complex, individual, time varying, dynamic system, this model has to be estimated for each horse individually and continuously during exercise. The time varying character of the system requires that the model is validated in real-time and re-estimated if necessary. This real-time input-output modelling allows determination of the component of the horse's heart rate which is solely related to physical activity.

Results and conclusions

The results of the experiment show that the measured heart rate can be related almost completely to the physical exercise of the horse during normal physical activity (trotting without any stress applied). However, when stress is applied during trotting by suddenly opening an umbrella, the component of the horse's heart rate related to the physical activity accounts for a significantly smaller part of the total heart rate, as can be seen in the Figure 1. This shows that the quantified component of the heart rate which is not related to physical activity can be used to quantify a negative mental status, in this case fear, of a horse during physical activity.

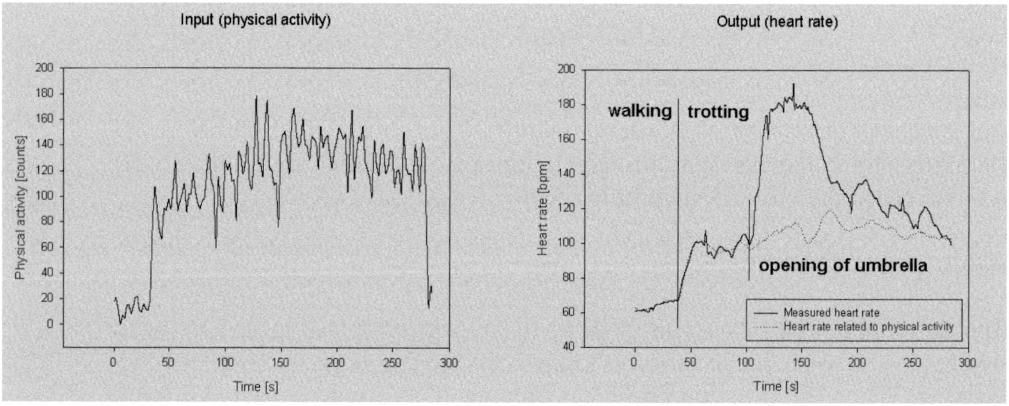

Figure 1. Measured physical activity and heart rate of a horse that was stressed during trotting by suddenly opening an umbrella. During normal physical activity (before opening of the umbrella) the measured heart rate can be related almost completely to the physical activity of the horse. After opening of the umbrella the heart rate related to the physical activity of the horse accounts for a significantly smaller part of the measured heart rate.

Serum cardiac troponin I and echocardiographic behavior of endurance horses in response to prolonged physical exercise

L.E.S. Michima, C.C.M. Bonomo, P. Miyashiro and W.R. Fernandes
Departamento de Clínica Médica, Faculdade de Medicina Veterinária e Zootecnia, Universidade de São Paulo, Brazil

Take home message

Serum cardiac troponin I and echocardiography did not detect severe myocardial lesions in horses after endurance races, but some echocardiographic alterations could be related to metabolic causes of disqualification.

Introduction

Prolonged physical exercise is associated to increases in cardiac troponin I (cTnI) levels in human and equine athletes, which may be related to myocardial injury or fatigue, and may also cause echocardiographic alterations, but the clinical significance of these findings must still be explained.

This study took place to examine whether prolonged physical exercise causes myocardial alterations, if these alterations have some influence on equine performance during competition, and whether there is a relationship with metabolic causes of disqualification, by means of cTnI determination and echocardiography in endurance horses.

Material and methods

Blood samples were collected from 30 adult horses participating in endurance contests, at rest (T0, control) the day before competition, within 30 to 60 minutes (T1), and within 90 to 120 minutes (T2) post-exercise. According to the distance raced horses were divided into three groups: G1 (races ranging from 120 to 160 km), G2 (races ranging from 60 to 80 km), and G3 (horses disqualified for presenting metabolic alterations). Serum cTnI determination was made using a commercially available immunometric chemiluminescent assay for human cTnI (DPC Immulite Turbo®). These horses were also subjected to B-mode and M-mode echocardiography, at the same times of blood sampling.

Results

Groups 1, 2, and 3 presented, respectively (mean ± (sd) serum cTnI (ng/ml)

- at T0: 0.13 (0.05); 0.18 (0.07); and 0.16 (0.03);
- at T1: 0.13 (0.03); 0.16 (0.06), and 0.12 (0.04);
- at T2: 0.12 (0.02), 0.15 (0.05), and 0.12 (0.04),

with the calculated 99th percentile of 0.30 ng/ml. There was no significant difference between groups ($p = 0.1244$) or sampling / measurement times ($p = 0.1843$), and only one horse (from G3) presented a value higher than the 99th percentile (0.32 ng/ml) in T1.

In opposition to cTnI results, alterations in echocardiographic variables were observed, among them a significant decrease of diastolic values of left ventricle in post-exercise ($p = 0.0019$) and an increase in interventricular septum thickness ($p < 0.0001$ in diastole and $p = 0.0057$ in sistole). However, there was no alteration of the myocardial contractile function, and there was no significant difference in left ventricle fractional shortening ($p = 0.4374$) or ejection fraction (0.3829). The trend in increased post-exercise cardiac output was influenced more by heart rate than by ejection volume. These alterations were more markedly observed in the first post-exercise measurement (T1), in animals that were disqualified by metabolic alterations, with signs of recovery to pre-exercise values in T2.

There was no relationship between cTnI values and place at the end of the race, distance, mean speed or any of the studied echocardiographic variables, as well as between many of the echocardiographic variables and the place at the end of the race, but for a mean positive correlation between the latter and cardiac output ($r = 0.38$, $p = 0.047$).

Discussion

Although it has been reported in human sports medicine that ultra-endurance exercise can cause myocardial lesion, the endurance physical exercise performed by horses, even those disqualified by metabolic causes, apparently was not sufficiently intense to induce the same type of injury. The observation of a trend of lower cTnI levels in post-exercise moments may be related to analytical interference, presence of auto-antibodies or even to increase in metabolism and degradation rate of the molecule. On the other hand, the echocardiographic alterations observed seem to be mainly related to decrease in preload, which could be caused by dehydration.

The findings of the echocardiographic variables and the absence of a relation with serum cardiac troponin I, seem to indicate that they have no apparent clinical relevance but for weak relation between disqualification and dehydration.

Conclusions

Prolonged physical exercise did not cause increases in serum cardiac troponin I, but caused echocardiographic alterations that apparently are not related to severe myocardial injuries in endurance horses, and these alterations might be related to dehydration, which might influence performance as a cause of disqualification.

Oxidative stress and exercise induced rhabdomyolysis in standardbred horses

E. van Erck[1], C. Loigerot[2], P. Lekeux[1] and N. Kirschvink[2]
[1]Equine Sports Medicine Centre, Faculty of Veterinary Medicine, University of Liège, Belgium
[2]Unit of Animal Physiology, Department for Veterinary Medicine, Faculty of Sciences, University of Namur, Belgium

Take home message

Exercise-induced rhabdomyolysis is associated with high levels of oxidative stress markers in poor performing racehorses. Measurement of lipid peroxide could be an interesting marker to identify horses at risk.

Introduction

Exercise-induced rhabdomyolysis is a common condition in sport horses which can cause poor performance. Horses suffering from recurrent rhabdomyolysis often need to be taken out of training and competition. Although equine exertional rhabdomyolysis can be multifactorial, exercise and diet management remain key factors to reduce its risks of occurrence.

Physical training and exercise induces the production of oxygen reactive species which causes cellular and tissue damage (Clarkson and Thompson, 2000). In man, exercise-induced oxidative stress contributes to the acceleration of muscle fatigue and muscle fibre damage (Sen and Packer, 2000). In the equine species, the occurrence of oxidative stress during exercise has been demonstrated (Hargreaves *et al.*, 2002; Kirschvink *et al.*, 2002). However, to our knowledge, the association between oxidative stress and exercise-induced rhabdomyolysis has not yet been investigated.

The purpose of this study was to establish if there was a relationship between antioxidant and oxidative stress markers and the occurrence of exercise-induced rhabdomyolysis. Oxidative stress measurements were performed systematically from the blood samples of Standardbred racehorses investigated routinely for poor performance or athletic follow-up.

Material and methods

Horses

A retrospective study of 142 cases of Standardbred trotters referred for athletic evaluation or poor performance were reviewed for this study. All horses were in training at the time of their examination and had undergone a complete clinical examination as well as a standardised exercise test on the same racetrack. During the exercise test, locomotion had been assessed. Respiratory endoscopy and tracheal and bronchoalveolar lavage samples had been performed after the exercise test.

Blood samples

Haematology and the activity of the muscular enzymes were determined prior to the exercise test (AST, LDH_0 and CK_0). The measurement of LDH and CK was renewed 60 minutes post-exercise (LDH_{60} and CK_{60}).

Antioxidant and oxidative stress markers were evaluated at rest, prior to the exercise test and included plasma hydrophilic (ACW) and lipophilic (ACL) antioxidant capacity, glutathione peroxidase (GPx) and lipid peroxide (LP).

Exercise test

The exercise test consisted of a 3000 m warm-up at a slow trot, followed by three 1500 m steps at incremental speeds (30, 35 and 42 km/h). The horses recovered at a slow trot over 500 m between each step. Speed was monitored using a portable GPS system (Garmin®, France). Heart rate was determined from continuous ECG recordings (Televet®, Denmark). A jugular venous sample was obtained after each step and blood lactate was measured with a validated portable system (Accusport®, Germany). The speeds at a HR of 200 bpm (V200) and at LA of 4 mmol/l (V4) were calculated.

Groups and statistics

According to the results of their clinical examination, blood work, exercise test, soundness and ancillary cardio-respiratory examinations, the horses were distributed into different groups. A group of 16 healthy, fit and performing horses was identified and considered as a control group (C). Horses with a history of poor performance and elevated values of AST, LDH or CK at rest or which displayed a two-fold or superior increase in CK activity 60 minutes after the exercise test were considered as having exercise-induced rhabdomyolysis (RM). Eighteen horses were included in the RM group.

Correlation between CK_0, CK_{60}, LDH_0 and LDH_{60} and antioxidant/oxidative stress markers was analysed for all 142 horses. Comparison of muscular enzyme activity, antioxidant/oxidative stress markers and athletic parameters between C and RM groups was performed using a Mann-Whitney test. The level of statistical significance was set at $P < 0.05$.

Results

The horses included in the RM and C groups were comparable in age (4.5 ± 1.7 and 5.2 ± 0.8 years respectively) and sex distribution was homogenous. In the RM group, all muscular enzyme activities were significantly higher compared to C group and the CK_{60} values reached after exercise were very variable.

Table 1 shows muscular enzyme activity in horses from the RM and C group, measured before and after the track exercise test. When considering the global database (n=142), there was a significant positive correlation between LDH activity and both GPx and LP levels ($p<0.02$). The correlation was less obvious for CK_{60} and GPx ($p=0.052$) or CK_{60} and LP ($p=0.07$).

Table 2 shows antioxidant/oxidative stress markers in horses from the RM and C group. There was no significant difference between RM and C groups for the antioxidant markers. However the oxidative stress marker LP was significantly increased in horses from the RM group.

Table 1. Muscular enzyme activity in horses from the RM and C group, measured before and after the track exercise test. Data are expressed as mean (± standard deviation) and (*) indicates the value is significantly different from that of the control group.

Group	TGO *(UI/l)*	LDH_0 *(UI/l)*	LDH_{60} *(UI/l)*	CK_0 *(UI/l)*	CK_{60} *(UI/l)*
RM	767*± 614	702* ± 244	730* ± 205	770* ± 1521	1175* ± 1510
Control	485 ± 570	490 ± 104	523 ± 101	205 ± 64	258 ± 101

Table 2. Antioxidant/oxidative stress markers in horses from the RM and C group. Data are expressed as mean (± SD) and (*) indicates the value is significantly different from that of the control group.

Group	ACW *(nmol equ.aa/ml)*	ACL *(nmol equ.aa/ml)*	GPx *(UI/gHb)*	LP *(µmol/l)*
RM	71± 36	22 ± 35	258 ± 49	90* ± 71
Control	82 ± 33	18 ± 8	282 ± 68	34 ± 26

The athletic parameters obtained through the track exercise test, were significantly lower in the RM group: V4 (35 ± 4 km/h for RM vs. 39 ± 4 km/h for C) and V200 (35 ± 4 km/h for RM vs. 40±3 km/h for C).

Conclusions

Horses with exertional rhabdomyolysis had decreased performances, which were reflected by low athletic parameters. The low V4 and V200 values in the RM group need to be interpreted with caution as other factors may markedly influence these parameters, such as training intensity and management, competition level and concomitant disease. Some horses in the RM group had concurrent conditions, such as mild to moderate lameness, inflammatory airway disease or exercise-induced pulmonary haemorrhage which may have further impaired their athletic capacity.

In man, oxidative stress causes the deterioration of muscle cellular membranes in inflammatory myopathies (Tews and Goebel, 1998). A previous study showed a positive correlation between LP and CK enzyme activity in horses participating in an endurance ride (Williams *et al.*, 2004). In our study, the positive correlation between muscular enzymes and lipid peroxydation and the significant increase in LP in the RM group shows there is a link between oxidative stress and the destruction of myocytes leading to pathological rhabdomyolysis in horses performing a moderate, short-term exercise. It is not possible without further investigation to determine if oxidative stress is a cause, an aggravating factor or even a consequence of repeated muscle cell damage. Nonetheless, results designate the LP oxidative stress marker as a suitable tool to evaluate horses at risk of exertional rhabdomyolysis. The dosage of LP could thus be integrated in routine blood analysis of sport horses and proposed in their follow-up during their training and competition season.

In sport horses, antioxidant supplementation during training can efficiently decrease oxidative stress markers (De Moffarts *et al.*, 2005). The potential positive benefits of antioxidant oral supplementation for the prevention of exercise-induced rhabdomyolysis should be looked into.

References

Clarkson, P.M. and H.S. Thompson, 2000. Antioxidants: what role do they play in physical activity and health ? American Journal of Clinical Nutrition 72, (Suppl 2): 637S-646.

De Moffarts, B., N. Kirschvink, T. Art, J. Pincemail and P. Lekeux, 2005. Effect of oral antioxidant supplementation on blood antioxidant status in trained thoroughbred horses. Vet. J., 169: 65-74.

Hargreaves, B.J., D.S. Kronfeld, J.N. Waldron, M.A. Lopes, L.S. Gay, K.E. Saker, W.L. Cooper, D.J. Sklan and P.A. Harris, 2002. Antioxidant status and muscle cell leakage during endurance exercise. Equine Vet. J., 34: Suppl, 116-121.

Kirschvink, N., L. Fi-Evez, V. Bougnet, T. Art, G. Degand, N. Smith, D. Marlin, C. Roberts, P. Harris and P. Lekeux, 2002. Effect of nutritional antioxidant supplementation on systemic and pulmonary antioxidant status, airway inflammation and lung function in heaves-affected horses. Equine Veterinary Journal 34: 705-712.

Sen, C.K. and L. Packer, 2000. Thiol homeostasis and supplements in physical exercise. Am. J. Clin. Nutr., 72: Suppl 2: 653S-669S.

Tews, D.S. and H.H. Goebel, 1998. Cell death and oxidative damage in inflammatory myopathies. Clin. Immunol. Immunopathol., 87: 240-247.

Williams, C.A., D.S. Kronfeldt, T.M. Hess, K.E. Saker, J.N. Waldron, K.M. Crandell, R.M. Hoffman and P.A. Harris, 2004. Antioxidant supplementation and subsequent oxidative stress of horses during an 80-km endurance race. J Anim Sci. 82: 588-94.

Treating the elite sports horse; can we determine withdrawal times from data available in the literature?

A.V. van Weezel Errens[1], A.H. Werners[2] and J. Fink-Gremmels[3]
[1]Lotlorièn BV, the Hague, the Netherlands
[2]Department of Equine Sciences, Faculty of Veterinary Medicine, Utrecht University, Utrecht, the Netherlands
[3]Department of Veterinary Pharmacology, Pharmacy and Toxicology, Faculty of Veterinary Medicine, Utrecht University, Utrecht, the Netherlands

Take home message

It was possible for 10 only of the 700 therapeutic substances for horses that were evaluated using literature data on pharmacokinetics and -dynamics to calculate withdrawal times and establish 'cut-off' values. Extrapolation from data of rat to horse resulted in large differences, hence adequate extrapolation of the elimination time of a substance from one species to another does not help in the establishment of 'cut-off' values for prohibited substances.

Introduction

Competition horses need veterinary care if they encounter diseases or are injured. As this may also take place during the competition season, veterinarians might have to take a decision to use a certain drug, with a long residence time, hindering the horse to participate in a competition. Other drugs, which may be less useful, but have a short residency time, may be used and hence confer no risk to the equine athlete to be accused for drug misuse and/or doping. To reach this conclusion, the responsible veterinarian would have to know what time span is required between application of the drug, and the excretion of the drug and its active metabolites to levels, that will not influence the behaviour of the animal, and/or its performance. At this moment there is a 'zero-tolerance' policy for all substances that are able to exert a pharmacological response in the horse, the only exception being certain drugs that are used in the therapy of gastric ulcers. In prescribed doping controls (see FEI regulations) urine or blood samples can be demanded directly after the competition, and the presence of pharmacologically active compounds result in penalties for rider and its trainer. Modern analytical techniques such as liquid chromatography coupled to mass spectrometry can detect drug molecules in concentrations that are unable to cause any significant biological response. Hence therapeutic intervention by a veterinarian, even under the best way of animal health care, can be identified, and the presence of these residual drug amounts will than be considered as doping, regardless of the biological activity of the compound under consideration. This policy was considered necessary to guarantee that in equine sports a fair competition is conducted, not only in terms of clean sports, but also in consideration of the economic interests involved in performing horses.

Positive doping samples as a result of therapeutic intervention cause negative publicity and a slur on the integrity of equestrian sports. Therefore it is important that regulatory bodies establish procedures that are transparent, but take into account the fact, that 'cut-off' levels exist, below which no biological activity can be observed in horses.

This research project aims to support veterinarians in their task to evaluate benefits and risks for a certain treatment, taking into account basic pharmacological and pharmacokinetic data and ultimately to estimate withdrawal time for sports, i.e. the EWT(s) (estimated withdrawal period) for therapeutic substances used in the treatment of competition horses.

Material and methods

This evaluation focuses on whether or not existing data regarding the pharmacokinetic and -dynamic parameters of therapeutic substances in horses provide a basis for establishing relevant and irrelevant plasma and urine concentrations (EPC, IPC, IUC). The EPC, IPC and IUC levels are calculated using the model as described by Toutain and Lassourd (2002), which links both pharmacokinetic and -dynamic parameters of a substance based on information retrieved after intravenous administration (independent of administration and formulation).

The evaluation is based on scientific literature (PubMed). Pharmacokinetic and dynamic information published until the summer of 2004 was assessed and the following parameters were used in the equations; total clearance (CL), volume of distribution (V_d), volume of distribution calculated by the area method ($V_{d(area)}$), effective dose (d), the dose-effect relationship Hill factor (H), steady state balance between plasma and urine (R_{ss}), concentration at which 50% of the maximum effect is reached (EC_{50}) and the effect at a given time point (E%), concentration at time 0 ($C_{(0)}$). When essential pharmacokinetic parameters were not provided, the WinNonlin nonlineair regression analysis programme was used to determine specific data from the calculated concentration-time curves. To calculate EPC, the lowest standard dose and the mean or highest clearance rates were used.

$$Cl_{total} = Q \times E$$

$$Q_{(ml/kg/min)} = 180\ BW_{(kg)}^{-0,19}$$

$$t_{½\ elimination} = \ln 2 \times V_d / Cl_{total}$$

$$EPC = (\text{standard dose per dosing interval}) / (Cl_{total})$$

$$IPC = EPC / \text{safety factor}$$

$$RA = IPC \times V_{d(area)}$$

$$IUC = IPC \times R_{ss}$$

$$E_{(\%)} = (E_{max} \times C_{(t)}^{H}) / (E_{(0)} + EC_{50}^{H} + C_{(t)}^{H})$$

$$D_{(t)} = C_{(t)} \times CL_{total}$$

$$WT_{(IPC)} = 1{,}44 \times t_{½\ elimination} * (\log (B_{(0)} / IPC)$$

$$C(0) = A \times e^{-\alpha.t} + B * e^{-\beta.t}$$

Where:
Q = cardiac output
E = extraction ratio
BW = 480 kg
EPC = Effective Plasma Concentration
IPC = Irrelevant Plasma Concentration
IUC = irrelevant Urine Concentration
RA = Residual amount

Secondly, the reliability of the extrapolation of pharmacokinetic and -dynamic data from rat to horse was evaluated. For those medicinal products used in horses with sufficient data to calculate EPC, IPC and IUC, the corresponding data in the rat were retrieved from the literature and EPC, IPC and IUC were calculated. Using the first three formulas mentioned above, the values determined in the rat were extrapolated to the horse, assuming that the volume of distribution of the substance was equal in both species. The values determined using the horse data were set at 100% and were compared with the extrapolated data. The reliability of the extrapolation was calculated.

Results

In total 291 articles provided data that could be used in this study. An IPC based on a Hill-factor could be established for only a few substances; the calculated withdrawal times are given in Table 1. For ketoprofen, meloxicam and vedaprofen no official Hill factor was reported. Hence the EPC, the IPC and the withdrawal time for the IPC were calculated using only the EC_{50} values (Table 2). The highest no effect level (HNEL) was reported in 7 substances (Table 3).

Table 1. Calculated IPC and IUC from substances with a known Hill factor.

Substance	Dose (mg/kg)	Hill factor	EPC (ng/ml)	Safety factor	IPC (ng/ml)	Withdrawal time $WT_{(IPC)}$ (hours)
Carprofen	0.7	1.56	3663.58	300	12.21	189
Clenbuterol	0.8 mcg/kg b.i.d.	0.32	1.08	700	0.0015	84.24
Clemastine	0.05	3.6	2.64	200	0.0053	56.43
Digoxin	4.6 mcg/kg	0.86	0.5	600	0.0008	22.37
Flunixin	1.1	0.89	612.37	600	1.02	18.45
Metocurine	0.01	4.6	80.75	200	0.4	29.25
Phenyl-butazone	4.4	1.03	4440	500	10	55.6

Table 2. Calculated IPC and IUC values for substances of which the Hill factor was not reported but tha EC_{50}.

Substance	Dosis (mg/kg)	EC_{50} (ng/ml)	EPC (ng/ml)	Safety factor	IPC (ng/ml)	Withdrawal time IPC (hours)
Ketoprofen (S)	1.1	33	120.76	500	0.24	14.52
Ketoprofen R/S	2.2	57 ± 9	308.6	500	0.62	6.7
Meloxicam	0.6	200	730	500	1.5	101
Vedaprofen	2	630 (94.5%)	250.7	500	0.50	30

Table 3. Substances with reported HNEL values.

Substance	Dosis (mg/kg)	HNEL (ng/ml)	Safety factor	IPC (ng/ml)	Withdrawal time IPC (hours)
Caffeine	2	2000	10	200	50.92
Carprofen	0.7	1500	10	150	120.7
Dimethyl sulfoxide	0.1			1000 (FEI)	65.15
Ibuprofen	10	200	10	20	8.58
Ketoprofen	1.1	400	10	40	5.14
Salicyclic acid				540 (FEI)	66.67
Theophylline	4.5 PO b.i.d.	10600	10	1060	35.13

Discussion

During the literature search it became evident that very little complete information had been published on pharmacokinetics and -dynamics of therapeutic substances in horses. Therefore calculation of withdrawal times and establishing 'cut-off' values was possible in only 10 of the 700 substances that were evaluated. Extrapolation from rat to horse resulted in large differences, hence adequate extrapolation of the elimination time of a substance from one species to another does not help us in the establishment of 'cut-off' values for prohibited substances.

Rules and regulations should allow veterinarians to perform their jobs properly. The use of cut-off levels would allow for treating veterinarians to adequately aid injured or diseased horses and still enable these horses to compete. To adopt the use of 'cut-off' levels of therapeutic substances it is essential that not only more research is initiated into the pharmacokinetics and -dynamics of medicinal products, but also the influences of exercise and feedstuffs on these parameters is considered.

Information regarding pharmacokinetic and dynamics of therapeutic substance in sport horses has recently been published in the Equine Sports Veterinary Manual. The manual enables veterinarians to estimate a (scientifically based) time post-treatment a horse should not be entered in competition, i.e. EWT(s). The EWT(s) is the minimum elimination time (MET) plus a safety margin, to allow for differences between horses such as breed, age, gender, size, metabolism, degree of fitness, nutraceuticals, other medications, recent illness etc.

References

Toutain, P.L. and V. Lassourd, 2002. Pharmacokinetic/pharmacodynamic approach to assess irrelevant plasma or urine drug concentrations in postcompetition samples for drug control in the horse. Equine Vet. J. 34: 242-249.

The influence of exercise and training on plasma acylcarnitine profile of Standardbred horses

Cornélie M. Westermann[1], Bert Dorland[2], Monique G.M. de Sain-van der Velden[2], Inge D. Wijnberg[1], Eric van Breda[3], Ellen de Graaf-Roelfsema[1], Hans A. Keizer[4] and Johannes H. van der Kolk[1]
[1]Department of Equine Sciences, Medicine Section, Faculty of Veterinary Medicine, Utrecht University, Yalelaan 114, 3508 TD Utrecht, the Netherlands
[2]Department of Metabolic and Endocrine Diseases, UMC Utrecht, Utrecht, the Netherlands
[3]Department of Movement Sciences, Faculty of Health Sciences, University of Maastricht, Maastricht, the Netherlands
[4]Department of Human Physiology and Sports Medicine, Free University of Brussels, Brussels, Belgium

Take home message

Assessment of plasma acylcarnitine profile in Standardbreds following exercise might provide a practical method to investigate potential disorders in carnitine metabolism associated with myopathy.

Introduction

It has been shown earlier that exercise in horses resulted in a decrease in free carnitine and an almost equivalent rise in acylcarnitine in gluteal muscle.

The current study evaluates the hypothesis that alterations in skeletal muscle carnitine metabolism during exercise and/or training lead to changes in plasma concentrations of acylcarnitines.

Material and methods

A longitudinal training study with ten Standardbred geldings (20 ± 2 months old and weighing 368 ± 45 kg) was performed on a high-speed treadmill for a total of 32 weeks. Training was divided into four periods:

- acclimatisation;
- training;
- intensified training;
- detraining.

In period 3, the horses were randomly divided into two groups: control and intensified training. At the end of each period, a standardized exercise test (SET) was performed. Acylcarnitine profile (34 metabolites from free carnitine to C18:1-dicarbon-carnitine) in plasma, sampled before and one hour after each SET, was assessed by electrospray tandem mass spectrometry.

Results were compared statistically using analysis of variance and values of $P<0.05$ were considered significant.

Results

Concentrations of C2-carnitine significantly increased in all SETS following exercise, whereas C3- and C4-carnitine significantly decreased. No significant effect of (intensified) training was found.

Conclusions

Also in Standardbreds carnitine forms esters predominantly with short- and medium-chain fatty acids. Plasma acylcarnitine profile seems to reflect skeletal muscle carnitine metabolism following exercise.